Unhappiness, Sadness and 'Depression'

Tullio Giraldi

Unhappiness, Sadness and 'Depression'

Antidepressants and the Mental Disorder Epidemic

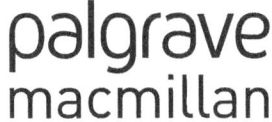

Tullio Giraldi
University of Trieste
Trieste, Italy

ISBN 978-3-319-57656-5   ISBN 978-3-319-57657-2   (eBook)
DOI 10.1007/978-3-319-57657-2

Library of Congress Control Number: 2017940344

Cover credit: FotografiaBasica/gettyimages

Printed on acid-free paper

This Palgrave Macmillan imprint is published by Springer Nature
The registered company is Springer International Publishing AG
The registered company address is: Gewerbestrasse 11, 6330 Cham, Switzerland

For my hugely supportive family, and in particular for Vlady, for the patience she has shown while I have been absorbed in writing this manuscript—in case I cannot express my gratitude in a future one…

Foreword

The great accomplishment of Tullio Giraldi's able and carefully considered work on antidepressants is to place these drugs in the context of the mental illness revolution.

As Giraldi shows, this revolution soon gave way to partial disappointment, because of the difficulty of translating its great hopes into concrete results. When the first international Symposium on Psychotropic Drugs was held in Milan in 1957, a good number of these drugs were already available and the main categories had been identified. The first tranquiliser, meprobamate, was already in circulation, as were phenothiazines, the first antipsychotics. Meanwhile, the sphere of "depression" was dominated by monoamine oxidase inhibitors.

From there, the number of antidepressant drugs increased enormously, and at present there are almost 40 available. However, the advantages of more recent drugs over their predecessors are limited, and their success is more often the result of advertising than of rigorously controlled clinical trials. Unfortunately, the pharmaceutical lobby has had a powerful influence on European legislation, and it's this legislation that guides the European Medicines Agency (EMA), the body that monitors drugs across Europe.

As a result, the law currently states that new drugs should be approved on the basis of their quality, safety and efficacy, and although these are all important considerations, they do not take into account what the public actually expects of new drugs: that they should improve on the old ones. In fact, simply adding the three words "therapeutic value added" to the current legislation would be enough to show up most of the 40 drugs currently available.

If you then consider that almost all the controlled clinical trials for approving new drugs are carried out by the pharmaceutical industry, it's reasonable to ask how we can accept this incredible conflict of interests. If European legislation only accepted clinical studies by independent, non-profit bodies, the range of antidepressant drugs on the market would probably be very different. And as Giraldi notes in this book, a significant shift in the way we use the various different "generations" of antidepressant drugs is currently underway. For example, Kirsch's studies have shown that, except in extreme cases of depression, there is no significant difference between the effects of antidepressant drugs and placebos. Even in extreme cases, antidepressants are only more effective because of the reduced effectiveness of placebos, and yet the vast majority of antidepressants are prescribed for cases where placebos would be just as effective.

It's important in this context to distinguish between the *disease* of depression and depressing *situations*. While the disease of depression is serious and therefore requires treatment, even when it is objectively difficult—given the lack of comparative studies—to choose the best method, depressing situations should not be considered pathological. If someone loses a loved one, has financial problems or is fired from their job, this naturally leads to a "depressed" emotional state. In such situations, people do not need antidepressant prescriptions but help realising that life goes on and that strength comes from within themselves. This is even more important when you consider that using antidepressants for extended periods causes withdrawal syndrome. That means that people who interrupt their treatment often resume it quickly in order to avoid symptoms that are even worse than before the prescription. That is why, today, people are advised to start not with antidepressants but with cognitive behavioural psychotherapeutic treatments, which controlled clinical studies have shown are just as effective as drugs.

This book suggests that we are still waiting for more effective and better-tolerated depression treatments. Unfortunately, for the moment multinational pharmaceutical companies seem to have deserted the field of psychopharmacology, deeming the discovery of new drugs both difficult and unprofitable. The sick, however, cannot wait, so it is now up to charities and the public sector to drive research programmes and develop new antidepressant drugs. And if the politicians and research programmers in charge of health agencies read Tullio Giraldi's excellent book, they must surely come to the same conclusion and support further research into treatments for depression.

Silvio Garattini
Direttore, IRCCS—Istituto di Ricerche
Farmacologiche "Mario Negri"

Acknowledgements

This book would not have been possible without the generous and unstinting support of Beneficentia Stiftung. I am profoundly grateful to them for backing not only my research but also my extended analysis of depression and other subjects in this work.

My sincere gratitude is also due to the Fondazione Callerio of Trieste, which supported my research and my work on this volume.

I would like to extend particularly heartfelt thanks to Dr. Maša Jović for the skill and dedication with which she has assisted me in the writing and editing of this text over the past few years. Her help with verifying the citations has been especially important.

I developed the ideas in this book largely as a result of many stimulating discussions over the years with numerous friends in medicine and experimental research. Attempting to list all of these people would inevitably lead to some unforgivable omissions. I will therefore limit myself to mentioning some of the institutions I have worked at in the course of my career, and which have provided me with extraordinarily stimulating academic environments. First, I should mention the Medicine and Surgery, Pharmacy and Psychology Faculties at the University of Trieste, where I have spent most of my academic career, with the exception of almost a decade at the nascent Faculty of Medicine and Surgery at the University of Udine and several short periods abroad.

I also have fond memories of my early forays into research with the Tom Connors group at the Chester Beatty Research Institute in London, and at the Bethesda Md National Cancer Institute and National Institute of Health. Here I had the pleasure and honour of working with the late Abe Goldin and numerous others.

Collaborating with colleagues from the Department of Mental Health and the local healthcare organisation, the Azienda per l'Assistenza Sanitaria no 1 Triestina, has also been an extraordinary experience. Their Franco Basaglia-inspired psychiatry and community care have left a strong impression.

Furthermore, I am delighted to have been able to contribute to the Slow Medicine movement in Italy, which is growing at such a rate now that it is even becoming influential at an international level, through associations such as Choosing Wisely. I am particularly grateful to all the staff and outstanding academic colleagues at the Department of Social Sciences in Health and Medicine at King's College, London, where I am currently a visiting professor, and where much of this book was written. In this hugely stimulating environment, I have been able to have many fascinating, in-depth discussions about often-delicate health-related subjects.

Finally, I would like to extend my heartfelt thanks to all the colleagues and students I have had the pleasure of working with in the course of my teaching and research. These experiences have certainly enriched me and I hope they have been mutually rewarding.

Contents

1

Introduction

The desire to take medicine is perhaps the greatest feature
which distinguishes man from animals.
William Osler

Depression: A Global Crisis'—this is the title of a document published in 2012 by the World Health Organization (WHO), which dedicated its 2012 World Mental Health Day to depression.

The contents of the document are alarming. The chapter entitled 'Depression: A Global Public Health Concern' shows how depression has become a significant contributor to the burden of illness in communities around the world. The WHO has also calculated that the total number of depression sufferers is approximately 350 million. In fact, a study carried out in 17 different countries found that an average of one in 20 people had reported an episode of depression in the previous year alone. The document also discusses how depressive disorders often begin at a young age and then re-emerge after the initial outbreak, reducing the sufferer's ability to function. Depression is becoming the principal cause of disability, and its incidence is growing worldwide: by 2030 it is set to become the main contributor to the global burden of illness.

© The Author(s) 2017
T. Giraldi, *Unhappiness, Sadness and 'Depression'*,
DOI 10.1007/978-3-319-57657-2_1

The Chap. 2, 'Depression as a Consequence of the Economic Crisis', contrasts surprisingly with this dramatic scenario. It underlines the importance of distinguishing between normal sadness and depression. It shows how adverse conditions like the death of a loved one, loss of social or financial status, frustration, disappointment and—particularly in certain cultures—personal humiliation cause normal negative psychological responses. In fact, in circumstances like these, it's a lack of response that should be considered abnormal, like the apathy often displayed by those suffering from mental illnesses such as schizophrenia or severe personality disorders. The chapter underscores the importance of differentiating between sadness, which entails "normal" responses to adverse events, and depression, which is marked by "ill", dysfunctional responses—even if making this distinction can sometimes be difficult.

This section of the WHO document is crucial, but it does not indicate how far the distinction between "normal" sadness and "ill" depressive behaviour could influence the overall incidence of depression (WHO 2012). There are numerous other issues that the WHO document does not address and that pose further serious questions.

Depression as a mental illness was relatively infrequent all the way up to the Second World War: it has only developed into an epidemic recently. What lies behind this growth? In fact, are we even right to see it as growth? The diagnostic criteria have changed, so could the increase in the number of cases just be because of these new diagnostic rules? Should normal conditions like unhappiness in the face of negative life events and an increasingly globalised world economy be seen as manifestations of mental suffering, and therefore included in the new diagnostic category of "major depressive disorders"? It is striking that today's psychiatric diagnoses are based only on the evaluation of patients' symptoms, and no longer identify cases of "mental illness" but only "mental disorders". These are also labelled "discomforts" or "conditions", but the term "illness" is avoided.

This is not the only disconcerting point to consider when examining the characterisation of depression in recent decades. In high-income countries such as the USA and the member states of the European Union, there is a striking parallel between the growth in the number of depression diagnoses and the increase in the consumption of antidepressants. One of the reasons for this is the successful marketing of a second generation of antidepressants: selective serotonin reuptake inhibitors (SSRIs). Their diffusion is impressive and it is estimated that between 1987 and 2002 the progenitor of this family of drugs—fluoxetine or "Prozac"—was prescribed to 40 million people in the USA, amounting to sales of more than 22 billion dollars.

While just as effective as their predecessors, these new active pharmaceutical ingredients cause much less pronounced side effects, yet a review of the scientific literature available reveals that, for forms of depression that are mild to moderate under the current classification, these new drugs only have a placebo effect, and even this depends on how effective the consumer believes the drug will be. A closer examination of these drugs also raises safety concerns. Certain, more severe forms of depression carry the risk of suicidal tendencies and, while it might be expected that pharmacotherapy would reduce this risk, studies have shown that these drugs actually make suicidality more likely in younger subjects. The risk is so great that it is actually mentioned on the SSRI labels and leaflets.

One of the most compelling justifications for using antidepressant drugs to treat depression relates to the theory of "chemical imbalance". According to this theory, mood disorders are caused by a chemical imbalance in the brain, and antidepressants work by correcting this imbalance. But more and more scientific evidence is calling this into question. The biological effects of antidepressants can certainly be detected in the chemistry of the brain but, despite numerous attempts to reduce it to simple mechanisms, we still do not understand what actually causes severe depression and why it responds to certain treatments.

These are some of the contradictions that appear when examining the scientific literature that has built up over the years about the phenomenon of depression, its treatment with antidepressants and its explosive growth. I will examine this literature further in the following chapters, and the reader will embark on a journey through the centuries, from Greek and Roman medicine to the birth of the modern scientific method, and from psychiatric and psychopharmacological treatments for depression to the most recent psychotherapeutic interventions, which are being used in combination with and as an alternative to pharmacotherapeutic treatments.

There are a vast number of scientific publications on depression and its treatment. Many credible and authoritative works have been produced that criticise the detectable distortions in clinical trials and contradict existing published results. In light of this, maximum care has been taken to base all content in this work on publications by qualified authors writing in the leading scientific journals. As far as possible, reviews, critical reviews and meta-analysis have been prioritised. Complex topics have also been handled with an appropriate level of detail and without forsaking any of the technical information necessary for interested, patient and attentive readers to gain a full understanding of the issues at hand.

References

WHO. (2012, October 10). *Depression: A global crisis World Mental Health Day.*   http://www.who.int/mental_health/management/depression/wfmh_paper_depression_wmhd_2012.pdf. Accessed 20 Mar 2015.

2

Melancholy and Depression

Though the doctors treated him, let his blood, and gave him
medications to drink, he nevertheless recovered.
Leo Tolstoy

It is generally accepted that the first term for a condition roughly
corresponding to "depression" was "melancholy", which dates back to
Hippocrates and the dawn of medicine in the Hellenic world (fifth to
fourth century BC). "Melancholy" refers to the basic foundation of
Hippocratic medicine: the theory that the human body was made up
of four "humours". This was also echoed by Galenic medicine in the
Roman world. In fact, this same idea was the theoretical foundation for
most medicine right up until the nineteenth century, when it was finally
abandoned because of the extraordinary advances in science and medicine during that period.

The foundation of the theory was that the human body was made
up of four humours: blood, yellow bile, black bile and phlegm. Each
of these was connected not only to the particular organ(s) where it was
produced (the liver, the spleen, the gall bladder, the brain and lungs)
but also to one of the seasons (spring, summer, autumn, winter) and

© The Author(s) 2017
T. Giraldi, *Unhappiness, Sadness and 'Depression'*,
DOI 10.1007/978-3-319-57657-2_2

one of the four elements (air, fire, earth, water). Each of them was also considered to have particular qualities (warm and moist, warm and dry, cold and dry, cold and moist), and it was thought that the prevalence of particular humours also gave rise to certain personality types or "temperaments": sanguine (blood), choleric (yellow bile), melancholic (black bile) and phlegmatic (phlegm).

Although humourist theory also took into account other factors—such as the environment, the season and the patient's diet and stage of life—bodily health was thought to fundamentally depend on the humours. Balanced humours (eucrasia) resulted in good health, while unbalanced humours (dyscrasia) led to disease (Cabras et al. 2005). In contemporary terms, this theoretical framework would probably be defined as "holistic" because it saw a patient's health as based on a range of internal and external factors.

The treatments derived from humourist theory were based on modifying certain dietary and external factors, as well as directly correcting the unbalanced humours in the patient's body. In a patient with a sanguine temperament, for example, ailments would often be attributed to an excess of blood, and physicians would therefore try to reduce the amount of blood with leeches or bloodletting. This practice in particular was used widely right up until the end of the nineteenth century, as it was easy to come up with theoretical explanations attributing most health disorders to excess blood, which should be treated with bloodletting. Evidently, such treatments could only ever have negligible positive effects, so serious illnesses would often worsen during treatment, and it seems that when patients showed little response, physicians would then resort to repeated and extended bloodletting.

As well as bloodletting, physicians would also drain other fluids, attempting to remove the toxic elements responsible for the illness. They would do so by administering vomit-inducing medication ("emetics" such as ipecac and emetic tartar) or laxatives ("cathartics" such as cascara and senna), by cupping[1] and by applying "poultices" containing irritants and blister agents. "Demonic possession", which was seen as a disease in itself, was the only exception to this because it was thought that it would not respond to medical treatment. Sufferers were instead left in the hands of religious authorities and exorcists (Greenstone 2010; Grube 1954; Lawlor 2012; Neuburger 1944; Belofsky 2013).

One famous historical example of these treatment methods was the case of King Charles II of England (1630–1685), who suffered an attack of convulsions and was treated by draining first 16 ounces of blood (approximately half a litre). This was followed by a further eight ounces of bloodletting. When this produced little response, he was subjected to an intensive course of enemas, poultices, herbal remedies and vomit-inducing emetics. He endured a total of 24 ounces of bloodletting before succumbing to his illness (Greenstone 2010).

The case of the US President George Washington was equally dramatic. When he deteriorated dramatically after an initial cold, his physicians treated him by drawing half a pint of blood (approximately a quarter of a litre), followed by a further 20, 20, 40 and 32 ounces. As his condition continued to deteriorate, bloodletting was combined with other treatments, including mercury salts, poultices, vesicants and an emetic tartar. He was then subjected to another 32 ounces of bloodletting before his death, at the age of 69, on the 14th of December 1799. His illness had lasted <2 days. During the most intense period of his treatment, a total of 3.75 litres of blood was drawn over 9–10 hours (Vadakan 2004).

These excesses show just how far therapeutic practices had strayed over the years from the original Hippocratic principles, which encouraged interventions that were respectful towards both the patient and the *vis medicatrix naturae*, or the "healing power of nature". Early Hippocratic physicians even believed that the body had natural healing mechanisms that could deal with serious illnesses. The role of medical interventions was just to trigger these mechanisms: they were never meant to be excessive or cause harm (Grube 1954; Neuburger 1944). There was also the equally respectful principle of *primum non nocere*, or "first, no harm to the patient", which has been maintained in various different forms down to the present day (Smith 2005).

Both of these principles helped to lay the foundations for the modern Darwinian evolutionary understanding of disease: namely that it is caused by an unfavourable combination of environmental and genetic-molecular factors, and that these same evolutionary drivers have also caused the development of healing mechanisms, which are normally very effective against illness (Nesse and Williams 1996).

These principles also helped to found the modern theory of "the natural history of disease", which examines the spontaneous evolution of serious conditions, how they are often overcome without treatment, and what this means for the efficiency and safety of therapy.

Returning to the theme of melancholy, the first description of this condition appears in the time of Greek Hippocratic medicine (fifth–fourth century BC). It was described as causing prolonged fear and discouragement and associated with the dry cold of autumn and the earth. It was attributed to an excess of the black bile (*melaina chole*) from which it takes its name. Since this time, terms such as "black mood" and "melancholia"—with its linguistic variants *melanconia* and *malinconia*—have become common terms for a depressed state. Because bloodletting was often associated with the administration of laxatives and emetics, this gave rise to the idea of "catharsis", or purification by releasing the moods or toxic substances causing suffering. The term was then extended to symbolic and psychological catharsis (Mattern 2011).

When considering the history of depression, it should be noted that, for many centuries, very little attention was paid to the mental illnesses and mood disorders of people from more disadvantaged classes who found themselves facing physical hardships such as wars and terrible epidemics. After the dawn of the Enlightenment, however, physical conditions began to improve for many, and more attention was paid to mental suffering. In English society at the end of the seventeenth century, the term "melancholia" was increasingly approaching the status of the milder conditions usually associated with the Victorian period, such as "hypochondria", "hysteria", "spleen", "vapours", the "English malady" and the "nervous breakdown" (Shorter 2013). This paved the way for the distinction between serious depressive disorders and milder but more widespread personal suffering. This latter category is associated with emotional and existential distress, and is a cultural, anthropological and medical construct which has changed continuously through the years (Shorter 2013). This is largely because the socially and medically accepted ways of describing personal suffering derived from familial and social hardship have changed many times (Shorter 1993).

Between the eighteenth and nineteenth centuries, different frameworks developed across England, Germany and France, largely because of the emergence of a contradiction between the somatic and functional theories of mental suffering. The first framed mental illness as a disease of the body, akin to many illnesses that were treated with internal medicine. This school of thought believed that mental illness was caused by a range of anatomical, functional and pathological factors that could be traced back to the nascent neurology of Willis and his followers. The second theory, however, traced mental disorders to a functional discomfort or disturbance. In the hands of Sigmund Freud and Emil Kraepelin, this theory would later develop into the fields of psychology and psychoanalytics on the one hand, and psychiatry on the other.

The psychoanalytical work of Freud has unquestionably played an enormous part in explaining how the mind functions, and is still hugely influential today, particularly at a cultural level. Freudian thought had a particularly strong influence on North American psychiatry after the Second World War, largely because of a number of eminent Jewish psychiatrists who fled to the USA from Nazi Europe. The influence of psychoanalysis on US psychiatry declined after that, however, giving way to the irrepressible rise of biological psychiatry, which relegated psychoanalysis to a secondary role.

Psychiatry, faced with the advance of biological psychiatry, seemed set to lose even its limited remaining role in medicine. It was largely only practised in mental hospitals, and played a small part in patient care in the absence of effective therapeutic tools. It thus became essential to create a system that would allow the effective definition and diagnosis of mental illnesses. In the event, this system was based on vital work by Kraepelin: his nosographic classification.

Although Kraepelin's work observing mentally ill patients in Munich at the end of the nineteenth century was hugely influential, he is nevertheless decidedly less well known than Freud. In fact, Kraepelin's work laid the foundations for essential psychiatric diagnostic tools like the American Psychiatric Association's *Diagnostic and Statistical Manual of Mental Disorders* (DSM). As the name suggests, it is a hefty manual that enables diagnosis by listing the assessment criteria for patients' symptoms. It was first published in 1952, had its fifth edition in 2013, and has been a notable success for the American Psychiatric Association (APA). In fact, it has sold almost half a million copies to date.

In Europe, the *International Classification of Diseases* (ICD)   was compiled by the World Health Organization (WHO) and published for the first time in 1948. It reached its tenth edition in 1992.

Over the years, the various editions of the DSM—including the recent DSM-5—have received much substantial, authoritative and well-founded criticism (Frances 2013a, b). The various editions of the ICD—which, unlike the DSM, cover *all* illnesses rather than just those of a psychiatric nature—have been embraced as useful classification and communication tools, aside from certain unresolved issues to do with creating diagnostic categories of psychiatric disorders.

At this point, however, it is perhaps useful to return to melancholy and depression to analyse how the relatively rare condition of serious melancholic depression became more frequent mild or moderate mood disturbances, and eventually became the modern "major depressive disorder" epidemic described by the DSM.

The creation of modern psychiatric diagnostic criteria was accompanied by significant changes to the definition of depressive mood disorders. Kraepelin's definition of mental illness categories was based on the careful observation of a large number of clinical cases between the nineteenth and twentieth centuries. It was a time when many people were waiting for the joint work of neurologists and psychiatrists to prove that mental illnesses were caused by organic lesions of the brain. Kraepelin's categories were based on the progression of the disease and the regularity of sets of symptoms (syndromes): these formed the basis for the subdivision of mental illnesses into two large groups. The first was made up of conditions characterised by thought disturbances that deteriorated over time, such as schizophrenia, then labelled *dementia praecox*. Conditions in this category required constant treatment, which could only be provided in mental hospitals.

The second category was made up of emotional and affective disorders, which typically manifested themselves episodically and could therefore go into temporary remission, allowing patients to return to everyday life. This condition was formerly labelled "manic depression", meaning depressive episodes that alternate with episodes of manic excitement. It has been given various names over the years, including "manic depression" and "cyclothymia", but it is now termed "bipolar disorder". Kraepelin initially defined a unipolar depressive disorder, "involutional melancholia", as separate from manic-depressive disorders, but abandoned the theory later. Kraepelin saw mania (characterised by elation, hyperactivity and tumultuous conception) and melancholy (characterised by a lowered mood and the inhibition of thought and bodily processes) as part of the same single morbid identity, the manic-depressive illness. He also saw that the depressive state could have different manifestations and degrees of severity, from the retardation of "melancholia simplex" and the psychotic symptoms of "melancholia gravis", to the rarest and most serious form, "delirious melancholia", which involved clouded consciousness and even catatonia (Bynum and Bynum 2011; Decker 2004; Engstrom 1991; Kraam 2002).

Sigmund Freud, a contemporary of Kraepelin, laid the foundations for an interesting alternative perspective. For Freud, mental suffering did not necessarily have physical causes, and was due to intra-psychic conflicts in the unconscious. Freud also saw that depression was often associated with anxiety, and it could be accompanied by physical ailments as well, such as a drop in a person's libido and energy. The idea that a depressive mood disorder could have external causes—which today we might call a *reactive* theory—originates from Freud's psychoanalytical studies, particularly those on mourning. Mourning is generally accompanied by transitory depression, which does not usually require intervention and is dealt with physiologically. This contrasts with melancholy, which is characterised by sadness, loss of pleasure and energy and a withdrawal from the external world. It is also endogenous and, unlike mourning, cannot be traced to unconscious psychodynamic adaptation mechanisms (Carhart-Harris et al. 2008; Flynn 1968; Lawlor 2012; Robertson 1979a, b; Shorter 1994; Spiegel 1976).

Overall, it seems that melancholy has gradually been relegated to a sort of theoretical and operational limbo, while the theory of two distinct, psychiatrically defined forms of depression has grown up in its place. In bipolar patients, depression is one of the two faces of manic depression and the patient passes from a state of manic excitement, which can entail dangerous behaviour if left untreated, to a state of depression, which in serious cases can even cause suicidal tendencies. These phases can vary in frequency and severity, and are interspersed with periods of quiescence. The severity of unipolar depression can also range from mild—characterised by a lowered mood and anxiety, which is often a reaction to life events—to serious, which is endogenous, cannot be traced to external events, and is often accompanied by suicidal tendencies (Craddock and Owen 2010; Paykel 2008).

The first half of the twentieth century saw the creation of a diagnostic framework for illnesses, which gave rise to diagnostic manuals that classified mental illnesses in social, clinical, medical, legal and insurance terms. The various versions of the ICD have not met with particular scientific or methodological criticisms, and have enabled the adoption of a shared terminology to define morbid entities across all areas of health. The various editions of the DSM have also been hugely influential because they have helped to transform psychiatry from a marginal branch of medicine into a modern specialism, which could forsake brutal and inefficient treatments and adopt therapeutic approaches based on new drugs. The development of the DSM made all of this possible, so its evolution merits a closer examination.

Note

1. An ancient Eastern practice in which small heated cups are placed on the skin. The subsequent loss of heat creates suction, which was meant to result in a curative action.

References

Belofsky, N. (2013). *Strange medicine. A shocking history of real medical practices through the ages*. London: Perigee Book.

Bynum, W., & Bynum, H. (2011). *Great discoveries in medicine*. London: Thames and Hudson.

Cabras, P. L., Lippi, D., & Lovari, F. (2005). *Due millenni di melancholia*. Bologna: CLUEB.

Carhart-Harris, R. L., Mayberg, H. S., Malizia, A. L. et al. (2008). Mourning and melancholia revisited: Correspondences between principles of Freudian metapsychology and empirical findings in neuropsychiatry. *Annals of General Psychiatry, 7*(9). doi:10.1186/1744-859X-7-9.

Craddock, N., & Owen, M. J. (2010). The Kraepelinian dichotomy—going, going … but still not gone. *British Journal of Psychiatry, 196*(2), 92–95.

Decker, H. S. (2004). The psychiatric works of Emil Kraepelin: A many-faceted story of modern medicine. *Journal of the History of the Neurosciences: Basic and Clinical Perspectives, 13*(3), 248–276.

Engstrom, E. J. (1991). Emil Kraepelin: Psychiatry and public affairs in Wilhelmine Germany. *History of psychiatry, 2*(6), 111–132.

Flynn, G. E. (1968). The development of the psychoanalytic concept of depression. *Journal of Psychiatric Nursing and Mental Health Services, 6*(3), 138–149.

Frances, A. (2013a). The new crisis of confidence in psychiatric diagnosis. *Annals of Internal Medicine, 159*(3), 221–222.

Frances, A. (2013b). *Saving normal: An insider's revolt against out-of control psychiatric diagnosis, DSM-5, Big Pharma, and the medicalization of ordinary life.* New York: HarperCollins.

Greenstone, G. (2010). The history of bloodletting. *BC Medical Journal, 52*(1), 12–14.

Grube, G. (1954). Greek medicine and the Greek genius. *Phoenix, 8*(4), 123–135.

Kraam, A. (2002). Essay review: The legacy of Kraepelin. *History of Psychiatry, 13*(52), 475–480.

Lawlor, C. (2012). *From melancholia to prozac: A history of depression.* Oxford: Oxford University Press.

Mattern, S. (2011). Galen and his patients. *Lancet, 378*(9790), 478–479.

Nesse, G. C., & Williams, R. M. (1996). *Why we get sick: The new science of darwinian medicine.* New York: Vintage Books.

Neuburger, M. (1944). An historical survey of the concept of nature from a medical viewpoint. *Isis, 35*(1), 16–28.

Paykel, E. S. (2008). Basic concepts of depression. *Dialogues in Clinical Neurosciences, 10*(3), 279–289.

Robertson, B. M. (1979a). The psychoanalytic theory of depression. Part I-The major contributors. *Canadian Psychiatric Association Journal, 24*(4), 341–352.

Robertson, B. M. (1979b). The psychoanalytic theory of depression. Part II-The major themes. *Canadian Journal of Psychiatry, 24*(6), 557–574.

Shorter, E. (1993). *From paralysis to fatigue: A history of psychosomatic illness in the modern era*. New York: The Free Press.

Shorter, E. (1994). *From the mind into the body: The cultural origins of psychosomatic disorders*. New York: The Free Press.

Shorter, E. (2013). *How everyone became depressed: The rise and fall of the nervous breakdown*. Oxford: Oxford University Press.

Smith, C. M. (2005). Origins and uses of primum non nocere—Above all, do not harm! *Journal of Clinical Pharmacology, 45*(4), 371–377.

Spiegel, R. (1976). Reflections on depression and melancholy: From myth to psychoanalysis. *Journal of the American Academy of Psychoanalysis, 4*(3), 279–300.

Vadakan, V. (2004). The asphyxiating and exsanguinating death of President George Washington. *The Permanente Journal, 8*(2), 76–79.

3

The Diagnosis

*The aim of medicine is to prevent disease and prolong life, the ideal
of medicine is to eliminate the need of a physician.*
William J. Mayo

Medicine made extraordinary progress in the twentieth century. This
is often taken for granted nowadays, but it is clearly recounted in
Le Fanu's *The Rise and Fall of Modern Medicine* (Le Fanu 1999). Here
Le Fanu examines the major achievements of medicine from the 1930s
to the 1980s, as well as the circumstances that made them possible. He
chooses 12 definitive moments from the period:

- 1935—The discovery of penicillin.
- 1949—The discovery of cortisone.
- 1950—Tuberculosis treatment with isoniazid streptomycin and PAS[1]
  (together with the identification of smoking as the cause of lung
  cancer).
- 1952—The birth of intensive care following the Copenhagen polio
  epidemic.

T. Giraldi, *Unhappiness, Sadness and 'Depression'*,
DOI 10.1007/978-3-319-57657-2_3

- 1952—The introduction of chlorpromazine in the treatment of schizophrenia.
- 1955—The first open-heart surgery.
- 1961—Charnley's hip replacement.
- 1963—The first kidney transplant.
- 1964—The development of medicine to prevent strokes.
- 1971—The development of a cure for childhood leukaemia.
- 1978—The first test-tube baby.
- 1984—The identification of *Helicobacter pylori* as the cause of gastric ulcers.

When Le Fanu pauses to examine the period after this, however, he discovers that the further progress which was expected because of the flourishing in both basic and clinical sciences simply did not materialise. He then goes on to analyse why the promises of the researchers of the period never became a reality. A sharp, attentive analysis of this subject was also carried out by Steven and Hilary Rose in their book *Genes, Cells and Brains* (Rose and Rose 2012). This penetrating work examines in particular why molecular genetics and genomics have produced such limited results for the fields of regenerative medicine and neuroscience. According to the Roses, biomedical research is expected to have an excessively large impact on clinical medicine because an enormous amount of funding is poured into it, which is expected to always produce proportionate profits. They also discuss the negative connections between the public and private spheres of academic research and its application.

The appearance of chlorpromazine an antipsychotic, has made it possible, for the first time, to effectively control the symptoms of schizophrenia with a drug. Practices involving physical restraint, which is therapeutically ineffective and lacks scientific grounding, were thus abandoned, helping psychiatry to become part of the modern face of medicine. Le Fanu rightly describes the birth and immediate experimental and clinical development of psychopharmacology as a fundamental of modern medical progress. I will go on to discuss this later and in greater depth, particularly in relation to depression.

Any reflection on health, mental health and health interventions is based on the existence of a well-defined morbid condition: the history of mankind is also the history of the significant events caused by illnesses. Only consider the example of bacteriology in relation to devastating outbreaks of the plague, cholera and smallpox, or the diseases caused by food poisoning—such as ergotism[2]—as well as those caused by dietary deficiencies, like scurvy, pellagra and cretinism. Serious mental disorders should be considered in a similar light: schizophrenia, manic depression, psychotic depression (which often entails symptoms of schizophrenia) and other major endogenous mental illnesses (without traceable external causes) should all be seen as serious morbid conditions.

It is important to note at this point that a full historical analysis of psychiatry is beyond the scope of this discussion. Some analysis is necessary, however. Conditions that cause serious mental suffering require serious and appropriate treatment, and it is for this reason that psychiatric hospitals have evolved. The contributions of numerous illustrious specialists have helped psychiatry to develop as a branch of medicine in its own right, distinct from neurology and other specialisms. In particular, the contributions of Philippe Pinel and Jean-Etienne Dominique Esquirol in France, as well as Emil Kraepelin in Bavaria and Eugen Bleuler in Zurich, cannot be overlooked. Nor can one forget the work of Jean-Martin Charcot and Josef Breuer, which was later taken up by Sigmund Freud, with far-reaching repercussions.

Given this history, it is hardly surprising that the American Psychiatric Association's (APA) diagnosis manuals go to great lengths to describe mental illnesses in psychiatric terms that put them in line with the growth and scientific progress of other medical disciplines.

The 1960s witnessed the great debate about the problem of psychiatric diagnosis. The importance of the problem is made crystal clear by Stanford Professor of Psychology David Rosenhan (1973) experiment. His study, published in the authoritative scientific journal *Science* under the heading 'On being sane in insane places', has become a classic (Rosenhan 1973). In his experiment, eight people of sound mental health were to visit a range of different hospitals claiming to have psychiatric disorders that required hospitalisation. These eight pseudo-patients included a psychologist in his early twenties, three older psychologists, a paediatrician, a psychiatrist, a painter and a housewife.

The group consisted of three women and five men. Having been told to keep the details of the experiment completely secret, the pseudopatients were asked to present themselves at 12 different hospitals across several states in the east and west of the USA. The hospitals varied considerably in size and included both public and private institutions with varying degrees of involvement in medical research.

The pseudopatients were to go straight to A&E, claiming to have heard voices. If questioned, they were to state that the voices they had heard were unclear, but they thought they had distinguished the words "empty", "hollow" and "thud". If they were questioned further, the pseudopatients were not to provide any other false answers, except in connection to their identity. They were to avoid showing any further signs of abnormality. It's hard to imagine how they were convinced to take part in the study, given that it called for them to feign mental illness and present themselves at a psychiatric ward without any assurance of getting through hospitalisation, treatment and discharge with no negative repercussions. Their bravery is beyond doubt.

In the event, none of the pseudopatients were uncovered: all of them were hospitalised on the grounds of schizophrenia. After between seven and 52 days, all of them were discharged with a diagnosis of schizophrenia in remission. The medical staff who encountered the pseudopatients completely failed to recognise their good mental health. Surprisingly, however, the other patients recognised it immediately. Right from the start, they insisted emphatically that the pseudopatients were not insane, claiming they must surely be journalists or professors because they were constantly taking down notes.

When the results of the study were published, many psychiatrists refused to believe this could have happened in a good hospital. In response, Rosenhan proposed an experimental protocol to verify his results. The staff at a nearby teaching hospital were informed that one or more pseudopatients would request to be admitted to their hospital in the next three months. They were then told to rate all the patients who appeared claiming to have psychiatric disorders on a scale of 1–10 based on how likely they were to be pseudopatients. Over the next three months, the hospital's medical staff carefully examined 193 patients. One member of staff identified 43 pseudopatients, a psychiatrist identified 23, while another psychiatrist and healthcare worker identified 19. In fact, no pseudopatients had been sent to the hospital.

It is easy to imagine the strong reaction Rosenhan's work sparked from the readers of *Science* and the wider American psychiatric community. Robert Spitzer, who had invested a great deal of time and energy into developing the new *Diagnostic and Statistical Manual of Mental Disorders* (DSM), was particularly disturbed. He wrote a detailed and meticulous 10-page article in the (1975) *Journal of Abnormal Psychology*, challenging Rosenhan's work (Spitzer 1975). Despite Spitzer's efforts, as well as many more recent challenges, the facts reported by Rosenhan spoke and continue to speak for themselves, and his work remains relevant today.

Let us now examine the circumstances that led to the 1952 publication of the DSM by the APA. DSM-I was 130 pages and described 106 diagnostic categories. From there, the number of pages and categories would increase dramatically. The second edition, published in 1968, listed 182 categories over 134 pages. After a number of important innovations, the 1980 DSM-III increased this number to 265 categories, listed over 494 pages. This then increased to 292 categories over 567 pages in the revised 1987 edition, DSM-III-R. In 1994, the DSM-IV listed 297 diagnostic categories over 886 pages. After a number of minor tweaks, this turned into the revised 2000 DSM-IV-TR. Then, after a 13-year interval, the DSM-5 was finally released, but not without significant difficulties and criticisms [DSM-I 1952; DSM-II 1968; DSM-III 1980; DSM-III-R 1987; DSM-IV 1994; DSM-IV-TR 2000; DSM-5 2013].

The DSM came about because of the drive to create a "universal" diagnostic tool that listed and defined symptoms or groups of symptoms (syndromes). The aim was to enable commonly accepted diagnoses for mental illness, which had been discussed before this time but remained elusive. Surprisingly, in the first edition of the DSM, the APA actually sidestepped the problem of how to define mental illness. In the contents and title of the DSM they referred to "disorders (disturbances, discomfort or mental disorders)", avoiding the term "illness" altogether. There were, of course, many limitations to this approach, not least the decision to consider only the presence of signs and symptoms in the diagnosis, along with the abandonment of any reference to psychology, psychodynamics and external factors that may have contributed to the mental suffering of the patient. The APA also chose not to consider causal internal and external factors and their interactions.

It's hardly surprising, then, that the expert APA panel that drafted the DSM had serious concerns not just because of these criticisms but also because of the problem of the reliability and replicability of diagnoses made using the DSM (Spitzer and Fleiss 1974). The numerous revisions to later editions, as well as the startling increase in both pages and diagnostic categories, show that the authors remained concerned that the DSM—despite countless modifications—might still be inadequate (Fischer 2012).

Despite these criticisms and limitations, however, the DSM has experienced enormous success—in the USA at least—and it is interesting to ask why. One key factor, beyond diagnosis, is treatment: it's important to bear in mind that psychopharmacology developed between 1950 and 1960. Each of the DSM's diagnostic categories effectively identified and defined a specific new "illness" (thus over 300 new "illnesses" were identified in the DSM-IV alone), and each of these new "illnesses" merited not only psychiatric and pharmacotherapeutic treatment but also research and new drugs. The DSM thus helped to identify new, unmet medical needs and potential drug consumers (Moncrieff 2009). Allen Frances's introduction to the (2013) DSM-5 offers an in-depth analysis of how the DSM has encouraged more and more mental disorder diagnoses. In fact, one of the original authors of the DSM grew so concerned by the scale of the phenomenon that he addressed it in his book *Saving Normal: An Insider's Revolt Against Out-of-Control Psychiatric Diagnosis, DSM-5, Big Pharma, and the Medicalization of Ordinary Life* (Frances 2013).

For the moment, I will return the focus to depression and limit my analysis to the more notoriously problematic aspects of the DSM. By employing a descriptive method that defined diagnostic categories by the frequency of symptoms or clusters of recurring symptoms, the APA essentially adopted an empirical approach. It was also an approach that lacked firm scientific grounding in intra-psychic mechanisms, external events and the inner workings of the brain at a molecular, cellular and systemic level. This has been pointed out again and again by numerous critics. There was particularly strong and well-argued criticism in Kutchins and Kirk's (1997) book *Making Us Crazy: DSM: The Psychiatric Bible and the Creation of Mental Disorders*. The authors' particular concerns centre on the DSM's pathologisation of daily life (essentially the DSM leading to the classification of emotions or non-morbid contingent difficulties as illnesses or disorders) and its almost complete disregard for the influence of social and gender problems on mental disorders.

Kutchins and Kirk dwell on two relevant cases to highlight the DSM's limitations: homosexuality and the mental suffering of war veterans. Homosexuality was defined as a mental disorder in DSM-I and DSM-II, where it was listed as a "sexual deviation" and categorised as a "sociopathic personality disturbance". This was equivalent to saying that homosexuals suffered from a mental disorder, and since the severity of diagnostic categories was not graded in the DSM, it effectively claimed that it was as severe as the other 181 mental disorders listed in the book. In the following years, the cause of homosexuality was fervently taken up by the sexual liberation movement, particularly on the West Coast of the USA, and a controversial issue like homosexuality naturally caused lively debate not just in wider society but also in the psychiatric world.

When panels of expert psychiatrists formed to draft the DSM-III, and in the absence of any new scientific evidence, the majority that had previously categorised homosexuality as a mental disorder evaporated. The DSM therefore ceased to classify homosexuality as a mental disorder. Kutchins and Kirk's book gives a detailed description of the circumstances that led to the DSM-III-R abandoning the "sexual orientation disturbance" category, which included homosexuality. It was replaced with the less severe "sexual disorders not otherwise specified, with persistent and marked distress about one's sexual orientation". Other controversial diagnoses like "premenstrual dysphoric disorder" and "masochistic personality disorder" were also abandoned (Kutchins and Kirk 1997).

Something similar happened with the psychiatric disturbances of war veterans. The first editions of the DSM had ignored records of the often severe mental suffering of soldiers during the two World Wars.

As early as the seventeenth century, "nostalgia" was known as the sol-diers' illness (Editorial BMJ 1976), and what would today be called "anxiety" and "reactive depression" had been observed and defined as "shell shock" during the First World War, then renamed "battle fatigue" in the Second World War (Shively and Perl 2012). The term "brain-washing" was then created during the Korean War to describe the suf-fering not only of soldiers but also of prisoners after being subjected to cruel interrogation (Kutchins and Kirk 1997; Jones and Wessely 2001). After suffering severe trauma in the Vietnam War, a large number of soldiers had great difficulty reintegrating into their home communities. Many veterans suffered physical injuries and mutilation, which were recognised by the state, but there was no legal recognition or care for those suffering serious mental problems caused by combat. Because of what Kutchins and Kirk describe as a sort of "diagnostic amnesia", their condition did not fall within the existing DSM categories. This meant that these combat-related mental disorders did not have any legal or medical status, could not be recognised by the state and were not cov-ered by health and social insurance.

Veterans, however, were able to muster significant public support through protests and political lobbying. Eventually, the authors of the DSM, rather than creating a new category for the mental suffering caused by war, included such mental disorders in the category "post-traumatic stress disorders" (PTSD). They were also covered by "anxi-ety disorders" and "dissociative fugue". The authors almost completely avoided referring explicitly to "war". In fact, in the DSM-IV the term "war" appears only nine times in more than 800 pages.

In the cases of both homosexuality and post-traumatic stress distur-bances, the APA's psychiatrists were not swayed by scientific studies but by public opinion and politicians. It was only because of this that vet-erans who suffered mental disturbances as a result of traumatic com-bat experiences were able to receive medical and social assistance. Even then, it was at the price of being categorised as mentally ill.

As the twentieth century progressed, the general perception of depression moved further and further away from the theories of Kraepelin. Freud's ideas evolved and were compiled and developed by Meyer in the USA. This not only laid the foundations for a new perspective on depression, it also coincided with the rise of North American psychiatry, which was beginning to overtake European psychiatric culture on the world stage.

Although Adolf Meyer was a Swiss contemporary of Kraepelin and Freud, he emigrated to the USA in 1892, and it was there that his work was to have an impact. Having abandoned the idea that mental illness could be clearly separated from personal circumstances, he became convinced that the concept of melancholy could replace depression. He criticised Kraepelin's definition of depression as inextricably linked to mania, finding it too inclusive, and he noted that many cases of depression could be distinguished outside Kraepelin's categories. He proposed abandoning "melancholy" as the term for a specific response to external circumstances and replacing it with "simple depression". Of course, Meyer's overall framework was far more complex than this, describing not just "simple depression" but a complex system of disorders and types of reaction which I will not deal with here.

Meyer's work was prolific and he coined numerous new terms. Some of these were quickly forgotten, such as "ergasiatria" and "ergasiologia",[3] but others such as "psychobiology" and "mental hygiene" were fully accepted and remain in use today. Nor was it just the *term* "psychobiology" that came into use; his notion that every patient should be understood through a comprehensive assessment of their biological, psychological and social characteristics has since been fully accepted. Meyer also believed that the depressive mental state was closely connected to the world of work and conceived of "occupational therapy", involving treatment for depression and other mental disturbances. He then practised this and proved its efficacy during his lifetime (Scull and Shulkin 2009).

There was another key contribution to the definition of depressive conditions before the APA's DSM, which came from the observation of soldiers' psychiatric problems, particularly during the Second World War. It became clear to observers that even people with no history of mental disturbances could develop serious psychiatric problems when exposed to traumatic events. However, it was found that even when an individual's threshold of resistance had been overwhelmed, successful psychiatric treatment was possible if they were removed from the traumatic situation. This reinforced the idea that, even in the general population, traumatic life experiences could cause mental suffering—even severe mental suffering—in sane people. Evidence at the time also indicated that treatment could be effective in these cases, and could even be administered without hospitalisation, and therefore without the stigma associated with mental institutions (Lawlor 2012). This picture was reinforced in 1954 by the landmark Midtown Manhattan Study, which was the first publication to demonstrate the role of psychosocial factors in health and mental illness (Srole 1975).

The first version of the DSM, the 1952 DSM-I, was designed to replace the *Statistical Manual for the Use of Hospitals for Mental Diseases*, which had set the standard for North American psychiatric practice ever since its publication in 1918. It focused on subjects suffering from serious mental disturbances in psychiatric hospitals, and its structure reflected the changes beginning to take place in the world of psychiatry. In particular, psychiatrists were taking on more and more patients suffering from milder mental disturbances. Their treatment could take place outside mental asylums and using less aggressive and invasive approaches based on psychodynamics and psychoanalytics. In this, you can see the influence of Meyer's ideas about the relationship between life events and the onset of depression ("reactive depression"), accompanied by anxiety disturbances. The distinction between "reactive depression" and "psychotic depression" was also maintained.

When the DSM-II was published in 1968, it distinguished "neurotic depression" (or "reactive/non-psychotic depression") from "manic depression" and "involutional melancholia", based on psychodynamic interpretations of internal conflict or the loss of loved ones. This approach was based on Freudian-Meyerian theory rather than the work of Kraepelin, but there was a radical shift away from this when the DSM-III was published in 1980 (Wilson 1993). There was also a move away from psychodynamic and psychoanalytical diagnostic criteria, which had prevailed until then, and towards Kraepelin's approach. As a result, diagnostic criteria were based on statistical analysis of the frequency of symptoms. This was an important move because it was part of an effort to overcome the many contradictions that still characterised psychiatry, and both John Feighner and his collaborators made particularly significant contributions to the DSM-III's new diagnostic criteria (Kendler et al. 2010).

Depression came to be seen as a unified disease, and all non-manic forms of depression were placed in a single category, despite the evidence indicating the difference between "neurotic depression" and "unipolar psychotic depression" (which is not associated with mania). According to the DSM-III, three criteria had to be met to diagnose depression:

(a) Dysphoric mood (feeling sad, a sense of hopelessness, etc.)
(b) The presence of five additional symptoms, including eating disorders, insomnia, a diminished ability to think, a sense of guilt, agitation, suicidal ideation, and lowered energy and pleasure in everyday activities.
(c) The continued presence of symptoms that have not been caused by concomitant diseases for at least a month.

According to the DSM-III, anyone who met these criteria should be diagnosed as depressed. No clear distinction was made between reactive and endogenous depression, however, because there were no criteria for differentiating normal month-long sadness from a morbid depressive state.

Robert Spitzer, who had already played a key role in the creation of the (1980) DSM-III, followed this up with the publication of his Research Diagnostic Criteria (Spitzer et al. 1978). These criteria were intended, as the name suggests, to be applied in the world of research. In the event, however, they had important clinical applications and played a key part in the diagnosis of depression. The amount of time for which symptoms had to have been present was reduced to a two-week period, and the term "depressed mood" was replaced by "loss of interest", both of which extended the diagnosis of depression to a much larger segment of the population. The symptoms necessary for a diagnosis of depression were also specified in greater detail. The serious limitations of the conceptual approach, however, were in no way attenuated, since there was no reference to the nature of the disturbance, its course, treatment and diagnosis. The relationship between normal and pathological sadness remained unsolved.

The DSM-III had a great impact on American psychiatry and, indirectly, on psychiatry right across the Western world. It defined a new entity, "major depressive disorder" (MDD), a unipolar disorder distinct from other depressive disorders, which could be easily and consistently diagnosed according to the manual's criteria. Some psychiatrists criticised the general approach of the DSM-III, however, because of the emphasis it placed on symptoms rather than etiology. They also criticised its failure to take into account other concomitant external factors besides mourning, and there was still no differentiation between sadness as a normal emotion and the condition of morbid sadness; this allowed for the pathologisation of people experiencing non-pathological moments of difficulty (Horwitz et al. 2007). All references to the neurotic and psychotic aspects of depression were also removed, as were any links to psychodynamics and psychoanalysis.

In 2000, the DSM-IV-TR was published, but there were no salient differences between it and its predecessor. MDD was still categorised as a unipolar mood disorder, which could manifest itself in "major depressive episodes" and was distinct from "dysthymia", a less intense depressive disorder. It also kept the category of MDD "sub-threshold cases", which was introduced by the DSM-III. These are essentially cases with only two of the nine diagnostic criteria for MDD. Mourning was still omitted, unless symptoms persisted for longer than 2 months. Substance abuse was also omitted, and the DSM-IV-TR still made no distinction between "mixed" and "manic" forms of depression. However, it's interesting to note the subcategory of "major depressive melancholic disorder", which relates back to traditional endogenous depression. This subcategory of depression was supposed to have internal causes and no relation to external events. It emerged because of some tweaks to the categories for identifying MDD, but it was limited in its application (Fischer 2012; Sanders 2011).

The DSM-III and, in particular, the DSM-IV and the DSM-IV-TR, have had notable success. They enabled commonly accepted diagnoses and allowed psychiatrists to play a significant role in science and medicine for the first time. They also helped to increase the salary and prestige of the psychiatric profession, which had been limited until then. Above all, they finally allowed psychiatrists to do the same as doctors from other specialisms: to diagnose and then treat illnesses in hospitals and outpatient facilities.

This coincided with the discovery of brain neurotransmitters, the introduction of psychiatric drugs and the birth of psychopharmacology and biochemical pharmacology. Many important drugs began to emerge, like antipsychotics, antimanic drugs, antidepressants and benzodiazepine anxiolytics, all of which are still essential therapeutic aids (Healy 2002).

In this context, every new DSM diagnostic category meant not only a new morbid identity but also an opportunity to develop specific new drugs to treat it. As a result, there was a unique alignment of interests between clinical psychiatry, which is obviously concerned with effectively treating as many mental disorders as possible, and the pharmaceutical industry, which aims to reap profits from the development of new medicines.

Endogenous depression is generally more serious and, because of ineffective treatment, usually used to result in hospitalisation. This picture has changed dramatically, however, because of two major developments in the 1950s and early 1960s. These were the definition of MDD by the DSM, and the development of psychometric scales for the quantitative diagnosis of depressive disorders, like the Hamilton Rating Scale for Depression (Hamilton 1960). The latter development has led to the unstoppable increase in the number of depression diagnoses, which has corresponded with the development of numerous new antidepressants. This is partly because it is now possible to follow outpatient treatment with increased prescriptions. In the following chapters I will discuss how the DSM and the unexpected growth of a market for new drugs have led to what can be described, in the USA at least, as a true mental disorder epidemic.

Despite the many criticisms levelled at it, one problem with the DSM has still not been given the attention it deserves. The many editions of the DSM have discussed the diagnosis of mental "disturbances" and "disorders" in legal, medical and insurance terms, and helped to incur the stigma of psychiatric diagnosis. The DSM's authors have effectively helped to transform the normal emotions and feelings associated with negative life events into a "mental disorder", a term they cautiously used instead of "mental illness". The following chapters will analyse how this came about, as well as its continuing consequences.

Notes

1. PAS: 4-aminosalicylic acid, also called Para-Amino-Salicylic (PAS) acid. It is a simple chemical substance which has proven effective in the treatment of tuberculosis when used immediately after streptomycin.
2. Ergotism: severe poisoning from food prepared with cereals contaminated by a small fungus called Claviceps purpurea (ergot). It has serious consequences for the nervous system and peripheral circulation.
3. The medical study of an individual's functions, activities, reactions and mental behaviours.

References

Editorial, B. M. J. (1976). Nostalgia: A vanished disease. *British Medical Journal, 1*(6014), 857–858.

Fischer, B. A. (2012). A review of American psychiatry through its diagnoses. The history and development of the diagnostic and statistical manual of mental disorders. *Journal of Nervous and Mental Diseses, 200*(12), 1022–1030.

Frances, A. (2013). *Saving normal: An insider's revolt against out-of control psychiatric diagnosis, DSM-5, Big Pharma, and the medicalization of ordinary life.* New York: HarperCollins Publisher.

Hamilton, M. (1960). A rating scale for depression. *Journal of Neurology Neurosurgery and Psychiatry, 23,* 56–62.

Healy, D. (2002). *The creation of psychopharmacology.* Cambridge, Mass: Harvard University Press.

Horwitz, A. V., Wakefield, J. C., & Spitzer, R. L. (2007). *The loss of sadness: How psychiatry transformed normal sorrow into depressive disorder.* Oxford: Oxford University Press.

Jones, E., & Wessely, S. (2001). Psychiatric battle casualties: An intra- and interwar comparison. *British Journal of Psychiatry, 178*(3), 242–247.

Kendler, K. S., Muñoz, R. A., & Murphy, G. (2010). The development of the feighner criteria: A historical perspective. *American Journal of Psychiatry, 167*(2), 134–142.

Kutchins, H., & Kirk, S. A. (1997). *Making us crazy. DSM: The psychiatric bible and the creation of mental disorders.* New York: The Free Press.

Lawlor, C. (2012). *From melancholia to prozac: A history of depression.* Oxford: Oxford University Press.

Le Fanu, J. (1999). *The rise and fall of modern medicine*. London: Little, Brown and Company.

Moncrieff, J. (2009). The pharmaceutical industry and the construction of psychiatric diagnoses. In *Journal of Ethics in Mental Health*, *4*(Sept. Suppl.).

Rose, S., & Rose, H. (2012). *Gene, cells and brains: Bioscience's promethean promises of the new biology*. London: Verso.

Rosenhan, D. L. (1973). On being sane in insane places. *Science, 179*(4070), 250–258.

Sanders, J. L. (2011). A distinct language and a historic pendulum: The evolution of the diagnostic and statistical manual of mental disorders. *Archives of Psychiatric Nursing, 25*(6), 394–403.

Scull, A., & Schulkin, Y. (2009). Psychobiology, psychiatry, and psychoanalysis: The intersecting careers of Adolf Meyer. Phyllis Greenacre, and Curt Richter. *Journal of Medical History, 53*(1), 5–36.

Shively, S. B., & Perl, D. P. (2012). Traumatic brain injury, shell shock, and posttraumatic stress disorder in the military-past, present, and future. *Journal of Head Trauma Rehabilitation, 27*(3), 234–239.

Spitzer, R. L. (1975). On pseudoscience in science, logic in remission, and psychiatric diagnosis: A critique of Rosenhan's "On being sane in insane places". *Journal of Abnormal Psychology, 84*(5), 442–452.

Spitzer, R. L., Endicott, J., & Robins, E. (1978). Research diagnostic criteria rationale and reliability. *Journal of the American Medical Association Psychiatry, 35*(6), 773–782.

Spitzer, R. L., & Fleiss, J. L. (1974). A re-analysis of the reliability of psychiatric diagnosis. *British Journal of Psychiatry, 125*(587), 341–347.

Srole, L. (1975). Measurement and classification in socio-psychiatric epidemiology: Midtown manhattan study (1954) and midtown manhattan restudy (1974). *Journal of Health and Social Behavior, 16*(4), 347–364.

Wilson, M. (1993). DSM-III and the transformation of American psychiatry: A history. *American Journal of Psychiatry, 150*(3), 399–410.

4

The Mental Disorder Epidemic

Modern medicine is a negation of health. It isn't organised to serve human health,
but only itself, as an institution. It makes more people sick than it heals.
Ivan Illich

The World Health Organization (WHO) is paying more and more attention to mental health. In particular, it is closely monitoring the individual and social repercussions of mental illnesses. To carry out its assessments, it has developed special tools to determine not only the years lived with disability (YLD), but also the disability adjusted life years (DALY). Depression has attracted particular attention in the last few years because of its rapid growth, so much so that the WHO made it the subject of the 2012 World Mental Health Day. It was entitled 'Depression: A Global Crisis'. It's probably worthwhile reflecting on the accompanying document of the same name, not least because of the esteemed reputation of the WHO (WHO 2012). This document refers to depression as a "global public concern" and describes it as a significant contributor to the global burden of disease (GBD), affecting a total of more than 350 million people worldwide. It also reported that,

© The Author(s) 2017
T. Giraldi, *Unhappiness, Sadness and 'Depression'*,
DOI 10.1007/978-3-319-57657-2_4

in the 17 countries surveyed, an average of one person in 20 reported suffering from a depressive episode in the previous year alone.

The WHO describes depression as follows:

> Depression is a common mental disorder that presents with depressed mood, loss of interest or pleasure, decreased energy, feelings of guilt or low self-worth, disturbed sleep or appetite, and poor concentration; moreover, depression often comes with symptoms of anxiety. These problems can become chronic or recurrent and lead to substantial impairments in an individual's ability to take care of his or her everyday responsibilities. At its worst, depression can lead to suicide; almost 1 million lives are lost yearly due to suicide, which translates to 3000 suicide deaths every day. For every person who completes a suicide, 20 or more may attempt to end his or her life. … While depression is the leading cause of disability for both males and females, the burden of depression is 50% higher for females than males, in both high-income and middle-income countries.

With regard to the treatment of depression, the WHO states that: "Depression is a disorder that can be reliably diagnosed and treated in primary care." This reflects the view of depression in the *Diagnostic and Statistical Manual of Mental Disorders* (DSM). Unlike previous WHO documents on depression, however, 'Depression: A Global Crisis' mentions bipolar affective disorder.

The WHO also deviates from the DSM and American Psychiatric Association (APA) positions in the next chapter, entitled 'Depression as a Consequence of the Economic Crisis'. It states:

> Normal sadness and depression. Under adverse conditions like the death of a relative, personal humiliation (especially in certain cultures), disappointment, loss of social status, even financial loss, a psychological response is expected and is, of course, normal. **Under these circumstances, it is lack of response that would be abnormal**, as is the case with the absence of response (apathy) often encountered in patients with schizophrenia and some patients with personality disorders. **It is, therefore, important to differentiate between sadness and depression, i.e. between an "adaptive" and a "dysfunctional" response to an adverse life event,**

even though this distinction is sometimes difficult. Both sadness and depression are expected during periods of economic crisis. In the former case, active labor market programs, family support, solidarity and psychological support are needed. In the latter case, in addition to the above, treatment for depression is also required.[1]

This part of the document is particularly important because it addresses the problem ignored by the various DSM editions: the fraught distinction between sadness as a feeling or normal emotion (for example, when adapting to difficult life events), and sadness caused by endogenous depression which cannot be traced to external events. This topic has been extensively covered in Horwitz's book *The Loss of Sadness, How Psychiatry Transformed Normal Sorrow into a Depressive Disorder* (Horwitz et al. 2007). Robert Spitzer, the architect of the early editions of the DSM, wrote a noteworthy introduction to this book. In it, he discusses the importance of distinguishing between the normal and the morbid reactive forms of depression.

The WHO document makes repeated reference to the rising number of depression cases. The WHO estimates that, by 2020, depression will be the second largest cause of disability, rising to the main cause by 2030:

Depression is a common mental disorder that presents with depressed mood, loss of interest or pleasure, decreased energy, feelings of guilt or low self-worth, disturbed sleep or appetite, and poor concentration; moreover, depression often comes with symptoms of anxiety. These problems can become chronic or recurrent and lead to substantial impairments in an individual's ability to take care of his or her everyday responsibilities. At its worst, depression can lead to suicide, a tragic fatality associated with the loss of about 850,000 lives every year. Depression is the leading cause of disability as measured by YLD (years lived with disability), and the fourth leading contributor to global burden of disease as measured by DALY (disability adjusted life years) in 2000. By the year 2020, depression is projected to reach second place in the ranking of disability adjusted life years (DALY) calculated for both genders and all ages. Depression occurs in persons of all genders, ages and backgrounds. Depression is common, affecting about 121 million people worldwide and is among the leading causes of disability, it can be reliably diagnosed and treated in primary care; fewer than a quarter of those affected have access to effective treatments.

This description of depression is much the same as in most other WHO documents since 2000. These documents are based on reviews published in respected scientific journals, and seem to use North American psychiatric models for the diagnosis of mental disorders. However, as other researchers have pointed out, this WHO document also underlines the importance of distinguishing between "normal sadness" and "depression": essentially between "adaptive" and "dysfunctional" responses to adverse life events (Horwitz et al. 2007; Maj 2008). The WHO emphasises that both conditions appear more frequently in times of crisis, which means more active measures are necessary in the labour market, along with support for families, solidarity and psychological support; antidepressant treatment is also necessary for cases of depression.

It's important, therefore, to examine more closely how depression affects the GBD. In 2010, a study comparing all diseases found that depressive disorders were the second largest cause of YLD, with depressive disorders accounting for 8.2% and dysthymia for 1.4%. Depressive disorders were also the main cause for the reduction of DALY, with major depressive disorders accounting for 2.5%, and dysthymia for 0.5%. The study found that, on average, more women and working-age adults were affected by depressive disorders, and that there were greater regional variations for major depressive disorders than for dysthymia. It also suggested that depressive disorders made a substantial contribution to suicides and cardiac illnesses (Ferrari et al. 2013).

A year-long study from 2010 found that depressive disorders were particularly prevalent in Europe, and that each year 38.2% of the EU population suffers from a mental disorder, which amounts to 164 million people across the continent. The most frequent were: anxiety-related disorders (14%), insomnia (7%) and major depression (6.9%). The study also found that mental disorders accounted for 26.6% of the total burden of disease, with depression as the biggest factor. This was a higher percentage than in other parts of the world, and the study also found substantial differences between different age groups and genders.

The authors concluded that one-third of the population of the European Union suffers from mental disorders each year, and that together with neurological problems they appear to be the leading cause of disease in Europe. They also found that only one-third of cases receive some form of medical treatment, showing that there are considerable unmet medical needs (Wittchen et al. 2011).

More generally, studies about the epidemiology of depression agree that its prevalence varies significantly across different regions and cultures around the world (Kessler and Bromet 2013), not to mention across genders (Culberston 1997) and more- and less-globalised areas (Bhugra and Mastrogianni 2003).

As a nation, the USA has a particularly high incidence of depression. A 1994 study by Kessler evaluated a sample of subjects from across the country, who had all undergone structured psychiatric interviewing based on the DSM-III. Almost 50% of respondents reported at least one mental disorder over the course of their lives, with 30% reporting one in the previous year. The most common complaint was a major depressive episode, often severe in nature, and with other co-occurring disorders. Affective and anxiety disorders were most prevalent among women, and only a minority of people who took part in the study had received any kind of treatment (Kessler et al. 1994).

The presence of mental disorders in the US population is particularly high. Noting this, Robert Whitaker decided to analyse this phenomenon in detail (Whitaker 2005), and he published his results in his *Anatomy of an Epidemic* (Whitaker 2010). Here, Whitaker notes that there was a progressive rise in the number of people suffering from mental disorders in the USA in the wake of the Second World War. He also rightly notes that the post-War years saw the introduction of chlorpromazine into psychiatry, which revolutionised schizophrenia treatment and was considered one of the greatest achievements of twentieth-century medicine. Other psychiatric drugs introduced in this period, such as anxiolytics, antimanic drugs and antidepressants, also played a key part in the therapeutic revolution in psychiatry.

A second revolution soon followed, with the development of a new generation of antidepressants: selective serotonin reuptake inhibitors (SSRIs) such as Prozac. These drugs had fewer side effects and were better tolerated, allowing effective depression treatment outside the confines of psychiatric wards. These major developments in psychiatric treatment should have reduced the prevalence of mental disorders; instead what followed was such a rapid growth in the number of cases that Whitaker was led to actually class it as an epidemic.

The WHO's evaluation of the spread of mental disorders is based on the global burden of disease, and the diagnostic criteria they used seem to have played an important part in the extraordinary results they obtained. In the case of depression, they almost universally used the DSM-III and DSM-IV diagnostic criteria for major depressive disorder, possibly combined with the ICD-10 categorisation (*The ICD-10 Classification of Mental and Behavioural Disorders* 2010) [ICD-10].

Whitaker used a different method for his analysis, which took into account the monthly Supplemental Security Income (SSI), or Social Security Disability Insurance (SSDI), which the US government provides to those suffering from a recognised disability caused by mental illness.

According to this data, 560,000 people were admitted to state and provincial psychiatric hospitals in the USA in 1995. Of these, 355,000 received a psychiatric diagnosis, while the rest were suffering from alcoholism, Alzheimer-induced dementia, or syphilis. In 1955, one in every 468 Americans was hospitalised due to mental illness. In 1987, the number of people who received SSI or SSDI assistance because of mental illness totalled 1.25 million, or one in every 184 Americans. People diagnosed with schizophrenia (over 267,000) accounted for the largest number of those hospitalised, and a smaller number were afflicted with manic-depressive disorder (over 50,000). An even smaller number were diagnosed with other mental disorders.

Although Whitaker recognises that the comparison of hospital admissions in 1955 with the provision of state subsidies in 1987 is methodologically flawed, he points out that it was based on official government data and is therefore a valid indication.

It's possible to analyse homogenous data by directly comparing the levels of SSI and SSDI provision in 1987 and 2007. Doing so shows that the number of mentally ill people receiving a disability allowance from the state doubled in just two decades, rising to 3.7 million, meaning that one in every 76 Americans was classified as mentally disabled. This is also a sixfold increase on the 1955 hospitalisations. In terms of the 1987/2007 comparison, Whitaker points out that the 1987 data is from before the marketing of Prozac, which was to have a significant medical and social impact. He notes that the major increase seen in 2007 occurred in spite of the introduction of this and a number of other second-generation psychiatric drugs. The number of people afflicted by major depression and bipolar manic-depressive disorder, which was relatively low in 1955 (a little over 50,000 were hospitalised), was also set to rise dramatically, reaching approximately 1.4 million at the time of Whitaker's analysis (in terms of SSI and SSDI support) (Whitaker 2005; Whitaker 2010).

Whitaker also focused on the ever-younger age groups receiving mental illness diagnoses; in particular, the controversial case of attention deficit hyperactivity disorder   (ADHD) in children (Whitaker 2010). I will not consider this further, however, because it does not relate to the matter at hand: depression.

Because depression cases are assessed according to diagnostic criteria, it's necessary to ask whether the increase in the number of cases is due to an actual rise in the number of depression sufferers, or merely the widening of the diagnostic criteria. As almost all studies on the prevalence of depression use the DSM-III and DSM-IV's major depressive disorder category, this seems the best place to start. In addition to the DSM, most studies also use various scales to measure the severity of depression. The most widely used of these is the Hamilton Rating Scale for Depression (HRSD) . Originally published in 1960 (Hamilton 1960), it has been amended numerous times since then, generally in response to a range of criticisms.

The number of depression sufferers has risen enormously in spite of the introduction of antidepressants, so it seems right to take into account not only the problems with diagnosis but also the effectiveness of antidepressants, and the questions of why so many more people are using them, and why they seem unable to reduce the number of depression sufferers.

It is interesting to note how, in general, therapeutic progress has been made possible by advances in diagnosis and in the physical examination of patients—particularly inspection, palpation, percussion, auscultation and the use of increasingly sophisticated tools, thanks to advances in physics and chemistry. The great therapeutic achievements of our own time are the result of a long succession of advances in diagnosis and semiology (the study of signs and symptoms) (Porter 2002). Examples include: microscopy and its applications for pathological anatomy and infectious diseases; the stethoscope; the thermometer; the sphygmomanometer; the spirometer; electrocardiography; the discovery and diagnostic use of X-rays; and clinical chemistry. As a result of such diagnostic advances, patients can now be examined using ever-more sophisticated techniques, and based on an objective understanding of the structure and function of the body and its fluids, organs and tissue cells. Advances in diagnostics have also paved the way for diagnostic imaging with X-ray-computed tomography (CAT), magnetic resonance (MR) and positron emission tomography (PET). Laboratory techniques themselves have become extremely sophisticated too, and now include molecular-genetic analysis and the analytical use of metabolism and illness markers, both of which have made significant contributions to medical progress (Berger 1999; Bynum and Bynum 2011). Because of these advances in diagnosis and laboratory techniques, it is now possible to objectively document any sign of illness, to the point where we can actually identify miniscule "anomalies" whose prognostic significance we do not yet understand.

In fact, there is a growing concern that these developments could have led to overdiagnosis. It seems possible that this could have caused the growing number of medical and therapeutic interventions we see at present, some of which are actually unnecessary and even harmful (Welch et al. 2012). This has contributed to the rise of defensive medicine, and a number of court cases due to malpractice (Studdert et al. 2005; Summerton 1995).

In this context, it's necessary to consider the concept of psychiatric diagnosis itself. After almost a century of debate and criticism, it is still a contested practice, accused by its critics of lacking a sound scientific basis, of medicalising and pathologising non-morbid conditions, and of failing to resolve the underlying ambiguities and uncertainties highlighted by the antipsychiatry movement in the 1960s and after (Pilgrim 2007).

In hospitals and outpatient facilities today, general practitioners and specialists arrange extensive and sophisticated clinical and laboratory tests for their patients, using the most advanced equipment and methodology. Psychiatrists, on the other hand, try to diagnose their patients by tracing their symptoms in the 900 pages and 300 diagnostic categories of the DSM-IV-TR.

Today, the term "depression", if not accompanied by further details, is almost universally associated with the DSM's "major depressive disorder". It's a phrase that, if nothing else, suggests a certain degree of severity. The WHO World Mental Health Day document, on the other hand, defines depression as "a disorder that can be reliably diagnosed and treated in primary care" (WHO 2012). It is probably useful, therefore, to examine how depression is diagnosed in the DSM-IV-TR.

It divides mood disorders into "depressive disorders" (unipolar depression) and "bipolar disorders". It also includes two further types: "depression induced by substances" and "depression caused by other medical conditions". It further divides "depressive disorders" into "major depressive disorder", "dysthymia" and "depressive disorder not otherwise specified" (which it divides into "adjustment disorder with depressed mood" and "adjustment disorder with mixed anxiety and depressed mood"). Further subcategorisations are also possible, depending on the severity of cases, the presence of psychotic or melancholic symptoms and post-partum presentations.

Now let's look at how "major depressive disorder" is actually diagnosed. The first criterion of the DSM is that "five (or more) of the following symptoms have been present during the same two-week period and represent a change from previous functioning; at least one of the symptoms is either (1) depressed mood or (2) loss of interest or pleasure".

Depressive disorders, therefore, cannot be diagnosed unless the patient has at least a "depressed mood" or a "loss of interest or pleasure". It is surprising, therefore, that nowhere in all its 900 pages does the DSM-IV-TR specifically define the term "depressed mood". It is immediately understood in a colloquial context, and it appears widely in psychiatric terminology and literature, but the DSM does not offer a specific definition of it. A definition can be found, however, in Hamilton's book about the psychometric scale for depression, the HRSD (Hamilton 1960). In the first question of the HRSD, he describes a "depressed mood" as a "feeling of sadness, hopelessness, helplessness and worthlessness". The problem with the HRSD, however, is that it should only be used *after* the diagnosis of depression, so neither the scale's definition of a "depressed mood" nor any of its other contents can play a part in DSM's diagnostic criteria. The DSM also fails to include a precise definition of "loss of interest or pleasure". This means that the diagnosis of depression is based on the judgement of the examiner, in the absence of shared objective criteria for a "depressed mood and loss of pleasure or interest".

The descriptions of the other symptoms are also quite surprising:

1. Depressed mood for **most of the day, nearly** every day, as indicated by either subjective report (feels sad or empty) or observation made by others (appears tearful). Note: in children and adolescents, can be irritable mood.
2. Markedly diminished interest or pleasure in all, or almost all, activities most of the day, **nearly** every day (as indicated by either subjective account or observation made by others).
3. Significant weight loss when not dieting or weight gain (e.g., a change of more than 5 percent of body weight in a month), or decrease or increase in appetite **nearly** every day. Note: in children, consider failure to make expected weight gains.
4. Insomnia or hypersomnia nearly every day.
5. Psychomotor agitation or retardation **nearly** every day (observable by others, not merely subjective feelings of restlessness or being slowed down).
6. Fatigue or loss of energy **nearly** every day.
7. Feelings of worthlessness or **excessive or inappropriate guilt** (which may be delusional) **nearly** every day (not merely self-reproach or guilt about being sick).
8. Diminished ability to think or concentrate, or indecisiveness, **nearly** every day (either by subjective account or as observed by others).
9. Recurrent thoughts of death (not just fear of dying), recurrent suicidal ideation without a specific plan, or a suicide attempt or a specific plan for committing suicide[2].

There is an important specification in Point E of the guidelines: "The symptoms are better accounted for by Bereavement, i.e., after the loss of a loved one, the symptoms persist for longer than 2 months or are characterised by a marked functional impairment, morbid preoccupation with worthlessness, suicidal ideation, psychotic symptoms or psychomotor retardation." Thus, if the "depressed mood and loss of pleasure or interest"—which are not more clearly defined here—last longer than two months, the subject is diagnosed with major depressive disorder. The DSM-5, however, did attenuate the diagnosis in bereavement-related cases.

A further important specification is the possibility of extending the diagnosis to children and adolescents. In this case, the "depressed mood" symptom can be substituted with an "irritable mood", which the DSM does not go on to define more clearly. Depression in children and adolescents is a delicate and complex matter, but it is a phenomenon that is growing at such a rapid rate that these guidelines deal with it in detail. This is based on meta-analysis of a 2005 (revised in 2013) publication by the National Institute for Health and Care Excellence (NICE), associated with the UK's National Health Service (NHS) (NICE 2013).

The issue of post-partum depression, however, receives little attention in the DSM, despite the severity of the problem, as indicated by the extensive literature review the University of Toronto carried out for the Canadian health system (Stewart et al. 2003) and the guidelines adopted in various countries (Haran et al. 2014).

What is so surprising about the DSM's description of the other nine symptoms of depression is that it appears to be based on a mix of psychiatric and layman's terms. It also makes no reference to objective scientific sources, instead using terms that can be interpreted arbitrarily, such as "nearly", "largely", "excessive" and "inappropriate".

Predictably, the DSM's failure to use objective criteria and tools has led to numerous diagnostic variations over time. Shorter, an established psychiatric authority, points out that psychiatry has seen many inferior diagnostic methods (fads) over the years, and analyses why this has happened more in psychiatry than in other fields. He observes that the twentieth century witnessed a revolution in psychiatry, which brought it closer to the realm of scientific medicine. In particular, he notes the appearance of psychopharmacology and the development of the dexamethasone suppression test.[3] At the same time, however, Shorter complains that these very developments have contributed to the rise of inferior, unfounded methods, and fuelled the growth in the number of diagnoses and prescriptions: "psychopharmacology is no exception, with the faddish neurotransmitter doctrine taking centre stage" (Shorter 2013).

Shorter's concerns are clear when he discusses the difficulty of psychiatric diagnosis and the unfulfilled promise that pharmacology and neuroscience could help bring psychiatry and depression into the world of scientific medicine. In this context, it's also useful to consider the problems highlighted by Krishnan and Nestler's review of the neurobiology of depression, published in *Nature* in 2008 (Krishnan and Nestler 2008).

Krishnan and Nestler's introduction refers to common questions about the high prevalence of mental disorders and the DSM's diagnostic criteria. They note that, despite the huge impact of depression, we only have a rudimentary understanding of its pathophysiology compared to other serious multifactorial diseases such as diabetes. They also admit that the diagnosis of depression is subjective and based on the presence of a number of symptoms over a certain period of time, which often occur alongside stress and anxiety. All these elements, they conclude, mean it is extremely difficult to identify the biological factors involved in depression.

The authors illustrate this with a table that outlines the characteristics of major depression and type 2 diabetes. About one in six individuals in the United States will succumb to clinical depression during their lifetime, and this is based on subjective-qualitative diagnosis. The chart also refers to the basic criteria of the DSM, and the monitoring of patients through standardised questionnaires. It shows the risk factors for depression as well, including stressful life events, and it also states that depression has a genetic hereditary risk of approximately 40%, even though the disease genes are unknown. The treatments it reports include: antidepressants, anticonvulsant therapy, psychotherapy and deep brain stimulation. Among these treatments, it notes that "exercise (physical) promotes recovery". In terms of pathogenesis, it records numerous conflicting points, which are followed by a question mark: hyper- or hypocortisolism (abnormal activity of the hypothalamic-pituitary-adrenal axis), alterations in neurotrophin signalling and abnormal hippocampal neurogenesis, deficits in brain reward processing, and abnormal cognitive styles (negative thinking).

All the known biological factors are listed, without referring to the problem of diagnosis and without a critical assessment of their clinical relevance. Even obsolete and widely criticised treatments like electroconvulsive therapy are listed, as well as heavily invasive treatments with little scientific grounding like deep brain stimulation. Psychotherapy, pharmacotherapy and physical exercise are also mentioned. The authors conclude that:

> … enormous gaps in the knowledge of depression and its treatment persist, and that researchers and clinicians must embrace the polysyndromic nature of depression and use a multidisciplinary approach to explore the neurobiological bases for the many subtypes of depression: it will be imperative to look beyond monoamine and neurotrophic mechanisms and expand knowledge about antidepressant pharmacogenetics. (Krishnan and Nestler 2008)

Krishnan and Nestler's review is a perfect example of the separation between clinical empiricism, with its psychosocial and psychodynamic methods, and the approaches of biological psychiatry and neuroscience (Rose and Rose 2012). According to Jablensky, the limitations of diagnostic criteria explicitly based on classification rules—which characterised biological psychiatry in the second half of the twentieth century—helped to bring about a conceptual shift in clinical psychiatry. This made it necessary to reconsider psychiatric practice, research and training and adopt suitable conceptual innovations (Jablensky 2007).

In light of these considerations, it's interesting to wonder what would happen if an experiment like Rosenhan's was arranged but for depression. In other words, healthy pseudopatients claiming to suffer from typical symptoms of depression: would doctors definitely identify them as imposters? No Rosenhan-style experiments for depression seem to have been carried out. However, a 2005 study on antidepressants used similar methods. It was published in *The Journal of the American Medical Association* (Kravitz et al. 2005). The aim of the study was to examine whether patients would be able to influence their doctors by requesting to be treated with antidepressants. The study was relevant because, in the USA, direct-to-consumer (patient) advertising is allowed for medicines.

The study was designed to include three situations: a request to receive a brand-name drug (i.e. a more expensive patented drug with a registered name); a request to receive an equivalent drug (i.e. a less expensive drug with an expired patent and a generic name), and no request. The study was rigorously designed, and based on the random assignment of three different requests by "standardised patients", who would simulate two depressive disorders (major depression and adjust-ment disorder with depressed mood). It was conducted across a sample of 152 general practitioners and internists selected from across the states of California and New York. The standardised patients were all healthy subjects who were carefully instructed to play two different roles in line with the DSM-IV diagnostic criteria. The first role was a patient suffer-ing from major depressive disorder. The subject (female) had to present herself as a 48-year-old, white, divorced mother of two. She had a full-time job, no physical or psychological problems or history of depression in the family, and was suffering wrist pain. She was to report that she had been feeling down for a month, and that it had become worse in the last two weeks. She was also to complain of a loss of interest and involvement in daily activities, low energy, fatigue, sensitivity to criti-cism, occasional poor appetite, interrupted sleep and waking up early. She also had to report occasional difficulty concentrating at work, tear-fulness, confusion, agitation, thought disorder and suicidal thinking.

The second role was a patient suffering from adjustment disorder with depressed mood and back pain. The standardised patient was a 45-year-old, white, divorced mother of two, who had agreed to early retirement rather than accepting a change of work location to another state. She was to complain about fatigue, stress, difficulty falling asleep three or four nights a week but without waking up early the morning after. She also had to report having reduced her routine physical activ-ity due to fatigue and fear of aggravating her back pain. Both types of standardised patients were also well versed in how to request treatment based on advertising they had seen on television.

The research results are impressive. The standardised patients carried out their roles excellently, and only 13% were discovered to be feigning a mood disorder. Moreover, in the major depression simulation, 53% of the prescribers agreed to the brand-name request, 76% to the equivalent drug request, and 13% prescribed antidepressants to patients who had made no request. In the adjustment disorder simulation, the figures were 55, 39 and 10% respectively. Therefore, not only were the (healthy) standardised patients not identified in 87% of the cases, but they were also prescribed antidepressants in almost half the cases where they requested them, and in about 10% of the cases where they did not request them (Kravitz et al. 2005).

The fallibility of the DSM as a diagnostic system seems evident and could certainly be behind the continuing rise in the number of depression cases reported. The diagnosis of mental disorders also goes hand in hand with their treatment, and antidepressant pharmacotherapy has, since its development, been spreading unstoppably, much like the diagnosis of mood disorders. It's necessary, therefore, to examine the role these drugs have played in the current mental disorder epidemic.

Notes

1. Emphasis added by the author.
2. Emphasis added by the author.
3. Test carried out by administering an anti-inflammatory steroid, which abnormally suppresses cortisol production in the depressed. It has not found universal application.

References

Berger, D. (1999). A brief history of medical diagnosis and the birth of the clinical laboratory. Part 1–Ancient times through the 19th century. *MLO: Medical Laboratory Observer, 31,* 28–30.

Bhugra, D., & Mastrogianni, A. (2003). Globalisation and mental disorders: Overview with relation to depression. *British Journal Psychiatry, 184*(1), 10–20.

Bynum, W., & Bynum, H. (2011). *Great discoveries in medicine.* London: Thames and Hudson.

Culberston, F. M. (1997). Depression and gender. An international review. *American Psychologist, 52*(1), 25–31.

Ferrari, A. J., Charlson, F. J., Norman, R. E., Patten, S. B., Freedman, G., Murray, C. J., Vos, T., & Whiteford, H. A. (2013). Burden of depressive disorders by country, sex, age, and year: Findings from the "global burden of disease study" 2010. *PLoS Medicine, 10*(11), e1001547.

Hamilton, M. (1960). A rating scale for depression. *Journal of Neurology, Neurosurgery and Psychiatry, 23,* 56–62.

Haran, C., van Driel, M., Mitchell, B. L., & Brodribb, W. E. (2014). Clinical guidelines for postpartum women and infants in primary care–a systematic review. *BMC Pregnancy and Childbirth, 14,* 51–60.

Horwitz, A. V., Wakefield, J. C., & Spitzer, R. L. (2007). *The loss of sadness: How psychiatry transformed normal sorrow into depressive disorder.* Oxford: Oxford University Press.

ICD-10. (2010). *The ICD-10 classification of mental and behavioural disorders.* World Health Organization. Retrieved April 15, 2015, from http://www.who.int/classifications/icd/en/bluebook.pdf.

Jablensky, A. (2007). Living in a Kraepelinian world: Kraepelin's impact on modern psychiatry. *History of Psychiatry, 18*(3), 381–387.

Kessler, R. C., & Bromet, E. J. (2013). The epidemiology of depression across cultures. *Annual Review of Public Health, 34,* 119–138.

Kessler, R. C., McGonagle, K. A., Zhao, S., Nelson, C. B., Hughes, M., Eshleman, S., Wittchen H. U., & Kendler K. S. (1994). Lifetime and 12-month prevalence of DSM-III-R psychiatric disorders in the United States. *Results From the National Comorbidity Survey, in Archives of General Psychiatry, 51*(1), 8–19.

Kravitz, R. L., Epstein, R. M., Feldman, M. P., Franz, C. E., Azari, R., Wilkes, M. S., Hinton, L., & Franks, P. (2005). Influence of patients' requests for direct-to-consumer advertised antidepressants. A Randomized Controlled Trial. *The Journal of American Medical Association, 293*(16), 1995–2002.

Krishnan, V., & Nestler, E. J. (2008). The molecular neurobiology of depression. *Nature, 455*(7215), 894–902.

Maj, M. (2008). Depression, bereavement, and "understandable" intense sadness: Should the DSM-IV approach be revised? *American Journal of Psychiatry, 165*(11), 1373–1375.

National Institute for Health and Care Excellence (NICE). (2013). *Depression in children and young people*. https://www.nice.org.uk/guidance/qs48. Accessed 12 April 2015.

Pilgrim, D. (2007). The survival of psychiatric diagnosis. *Social Science and Medicine, 65*(3), 536–547.

Porter, R. (2002). *Blood and guts: A short history of medicine*. London: Allen Lane.

Rose, S., & Rose, H. (2012). *Gene, cells and brains: Bioscience's promethean promises of the new biology*. London: Verso.

Shorter, E. (2013). Psychiatry and fads: Why is this field different from all other fields? *Canadian Journal of Psychiatry, 58*(10), 555–559.

Stewart, D. E., Robertson, E., Dennis, C-L., Grace, S. L., & Wallington, T. (2003). *Toronto public health, university health network women's health program*. http://www.who.int/mental_health/prevention/suicide/lit_review_post-partum_depression.pdf. Accessed March 20 2015.

Studdert, M., Mello, M. M., Sage, W. M., DesRoches, C. M., Peugh, J., Zapert, K., & Brennan, T. A. (2005). Defensive medicine among high-risk specialist physicians in a volatile malpractice enviroment. *Journal of the American Medical Association, 293*(21), 2609–2617.

Summerton, N. (1995). Positive and negative factors in defensive medicine: A questionnaire study of general practitioners. *British Medical Journal, 310*(6971), 27–29.

Welch, H. G., Schwartz, L., & Woloshin, S. (2012). *Overdiagnosed: Making people sick in the pursuit of health*. Boston: Beacon Press.

Whitaker, R. (2005). Anatomy of an epidemic: Psychiatric drugs and the astonishing rise of mental illness in America. *Ethical Human Psychology and Psychiatry, 7*(1), 23–35.

Whitaker, R. (2010). *Anatomy of an epidemic: Psychiatric drugs and the astonishing rise of mental illness in America*. New York: Crown Publishing Group.

WHO. (2012). *Depression: A global crisis world mental health day, October 10 2012*. http://www.who.int/mental_health/management/depression/wfmh_paper_depression_wmhd_2012.pdf Accessed March 20 2015.

Wittchen, H. U., Jacobi, F., Rehm, J., Gustavsson, A., Svensson, M., Jönsson, B., Olesen, J., Allgulander, C., Alonso, J., Faravelli, C., Fratiglioni, L., Jennum, P., Lieb, R., Maercker, A., van Os, J., Preisig, M., Salvador-Carulla, L., Simon, R., & Steinhausen, H. C. (2011). The size and burden of mental disorders and other disorders of the brain in Europe 2010. *European Neuropsychopharmacology, 21*(9), 655–679.

-

5

Early Treatments

When a lot of remedies are suggested for a disease, that means
it cannot be cured.
Anton Chekhov

Ever since Greek and Roman medicine, both organic and inorganic substances have been used in therapy. They have formed the basis for numerous pharmacopoeias[1] and have thereby been included in the medicinal remedies prescribed by doctors, dispensed by pharmacists and taken by patients. Over the years, many of these remedies proved ineffective and were abandoned. They were often condemned as fads, which Shorter has also complained about in the context of psychiatric diagnosis (Shorter 2013). As a result, many new and eagerly anticipated treatments were abandoned as useless, perhaps being rediscovered later only to be dismissed again.

Looking back at the history of pharmacology from a modern perspective, it seems that of all the natural remedies prepared by pharmacists, from the time of Hippocrates up to the eighteenth century, the active and effective ones (even by modern standards) were made from notoriously toxic plants. These plants, called "officinals", contain potent active

© The Author(s) 2017
T. Giraldi, *Unhappiness, Sadness and 'Depression'*,
DOI 10.1007/978-3-319-57657-2_5

ingredients, which in their purified form are still important—even indispensable—in modern medicine.

Let's consider one of the most well known: opium. Morphine and the other alkaloids it contains have significant effects on the central nervous system and the brain. Opium's usefulness for reducing pain has long been known, and morphine is still the benchmark for new analgesics. The psychotropic effects of opium have also been known for many centuries. As a result, opium has often been used not only to reduce pain, but also to induce a subjective sense of wellbeing in patients suffering from serious illnesses.

Since the days of Galen, physicians have used significant amounts of opium (as well as smaller quantities of other medicinal plants) to prepare an elixir[2] called theriaca or *mithridatum*. It was prescribed and deemed effective against several diseases, and remained a fixture of European pharmacopoeia until the nineteenth century (Norton 2006). Its popularity can be largely attributed to opium, which can alleviate the milder symptoms—like coughing and diarrhoea—of many serious illnesses such as tuberculosis and cholera.

Advances in the natural sciences, combined with centuries of exploration, have made the systematic study of medicinal plants possible. With its leading scientists and its extraordinary collection of medicinal plants from all over the world, Kew Gardens in London is an excellent example of this. Research at institutions like Kew has led to the identification of many active ingredients, including: digitalis, quinine, atropine, physostigmine, pilocarpine, scopolamine, curare, ephedrine, caffeine and methylxanthines, vitamins such as vitamin C and niacin, the anticancer vinca alkaloids and taxanes, and the new antimalarial artemisinin (Weatherall 1990).

The active substances contained in fungi (*Psilocybe*, psilocybin) and cacti (*Peyote*, mescaline) are intensely hallucinogenic (psychedelic) , and anthropological and ethnopharmacological studies have described their shamanic and ritual use (Abraham et al. 1996). For many centuries, the Andean people chewed coca leaves, containing cocaine, both for ritual purposes and to stave off the fatigue caused by agricultural labour in the mountains. The psychotropic effects of cannabis and hashish, caused by their tetrahydrocannabinol content, have also long been known (Zuardi 2006), as have the hallucinogenic effects of mandrake, caused by scopolamine (Crocq 2007). In Europe, the contamination of cereals by ergot has caused many severe food poisoning epidemics over the centuries. The active substance here was ergotamine, which caused ergotism or "St. Anthony's Fire" (Meggs 2009). Less serious cases were characterised by behavioural disorders and problems with the central nervous system. Some scholars even claim ergot poisoning led to the accusations of witchcraft in the infamous Salem witch trials of 1692 (Spanos and Gottlieb 1976; Matossian 1982).

While plants have contributed much to other areas of medicine, historically they have played very little part in the pharmacotherapy of mental disorders. In fact, because of addiction and substance abuse, they have actually caused many negative phenomena.

The study of electrical phenomena led to much more important historical developments in the treatment of nervous disorders. At the end of the eighteenth century, Luigi Galvani (1737–1798) used frogs to show that the electrical stimulation of nerves leads to muscle contraction. This gave rise to the term "animal electricity" , which is still inextricably linked to Galvani, along with the fascinating theory that there is a connection between life and electricity. Galvani's work was quickly embraced by the scientific community of the time, and it was soon enriched by new developments in the field of electricity, such as electrostatic generators, induction coils and Alessandro Volta's invention of the first electric battery.

Galvani's association of electricity with the nerves gave rise to the idea that electrical machines could be used to treat certain nervous disorders such as the "English malady" and spleen, which were supposedly prevalent among the English upper classes of the late-eighteenth and early-nineteenth centuries. "Faradism" developed and along with it "faradic treatment", which used extremely low-powered electrostatic generators, together with mild electric impulses from small Ruhmkorff induction coils. These Ruhmkorff coils—often housed in elegant, lacquered wood cabinets—were connected to crank- or battery-operated electrical components, which were, in turn, connected to brass cylindrical electrodes that were applied to the body.

The rise of electrical machinery and the idea that animal electricity was the basis of life helped to inspire Mary Shelley's 1818 work

Frankenstein; or The Modern Prometheus. In it, the protagonist, Victor Frankenstein, steals body parts from cemeteries and runs electricity through them to create life. Ignoring for a moment the complications the poor creature encounters, Shelley broadly seems to accept the widespread idea that electricity was connected with life, and that it could even infuse an inanimate body with life.

In hindsight, the inefficiency of electrotherapy for treating nervous disorders seems evident, and the practice was soon abandoned. Before long, electrotherapy instruments were relegated to the status of collectors' items. Two centuries later, however, they began to reappear, because of the controversial practice of electroconvulsive therapy (Shorter and Healy 2007) and, more recently, vagus nerve stimulation and deep brain stimulation (Basford 2001; Gilman 2008; Schwalb and Hamani 2008).

It wasn't just the study of electricity that was progressing during the eighteenth and nineteenth centuries: many developments were also made in the field of magnetism. While curious experimenters and clinicians occupied themselves with electrostatic generators, batteries and induction coils, other researchers were studying the effects of magnets on living organisms. One such researcher was Franz Anton Mesmer (1734–1815), a lively Viennese physician who gained considerable fame for his therapeutic successes at the end of the eighteenth century. His treatment sessions took a decidedly curious form, known as 'mesmerism': he would get several patients to hold hands in a chain, all with their bare feet immersed in tubs of water. Mesmer and his assistants would then move between the patients and the crowd of onlookers, carrying magnetised metal bars, which they applied to the sick. Typically, the subjects were suffering from "nervous" disorders (neurasthenia, neurosis or hysteria, with their possible somatic manifestations), and for many the treatment attenuated or cleared their symptoms.

Mesmer became well known and his therapeutic sessions turned into popular social events. He befriended important and celebrated figures of the time, including Baroness Maria Anna von Bosch, Baron Elias Wiksel (who recovered from suffocation anxiety, which included spasms in the pharynx) and Wolfgang Amadeus Mozart, who later referred to mesmerism in a comic scene in the first act of *Così fan tutte.*

However, his many successes were also accompanied by therapeutic failures and scandals, which forced Mesmer to leave Vienna (Forrest 2002). He moved to Paris, where he successfully resumed his work, but again his achievements were overshadowed by numerous doubts and criticisms. His many failures even led to doubts about his apparent successes. Two scientific committees of the luminaries of the age—including Benjamin Franklin—were formed to determine whether Mesmer's apparent achievements with animal magnetism were real. The committees carried out a serious, in-depth investigation with clear, decisive results: the therapeutic effects of Mesmer's treatment were not linked to magnets or animal magnetism, but were instead caused by auto-suggestion (Kihlstrom 2002).

Just as animal electricity had proved ineffective in therapy, so too did animal magnetism. But there was a difference. Whereas electrotherapy was shown to be ineffective as a treatment and promptly disappeared, animal magnetism became associated with mesmerism, which survived and became synonymous with the power of suggestion. Mesmerism laid the foundations for James Braid's (1795–1860) study of the power of suggestion and medical hypnosis. He went on to coin the term "hypnosis" in 1842. Today the term "mesmerise" still means to capture the attention of a person and induce a hypnotic state. Mesmerism also demonstrated that an ineffective treatment can produce clinical responses if done suggestively with impressionable subjects, which is a prime example of what would come to be known as the "placebo effect".

A less well-known case from the same period was that of the North American doctor Elisha Perkins (1741–1799). He invented the "tractor", a pointed metal rod which could treat a huge variety of diseases when passed over the patient. Perkins' therapeutic successes brought him widespread fame and his tractors even found their way to England, where they met with initial success. Eventually, however, they were subjected to the scrutiny of one John Haygarth (1740–1827). Haygarth was unconvinced by them and decided to determine their effectiveness by using fake tractors, made of wood rather than metal, on patients. He published his results in the book *Of the imagination, as a cause and as a cure of disorders of the body: exemplified by fictitious tractors, and epidemical convulsions* (Haygarth 1800). The book showed how the fake tractors were just as effective as the real ones, and it was the first work to effectively demonstrate the placebo effect (Booth 2005).

Serious and rigorous investigations, like the inquiry into mesmerism or Haygarth's work on Perkins' tractors, showed how many ineffective treatments were based on the power of suggestion, or simply on pure quackery (Bethard 2004). They also showed that it was necessary to develop specific methods for distinguishing real therapeutic action from the placebo effect. These were only clearly defined and fully applied in the second half of the twentieth century (Shorter 2011).

Surgery is a vital part of modern medical practice, and it achieved undisputed therapeutic success after the introduction of anaesthetics, asepsis and antiseptics. But unsurprisingly there have been many attempts over the years to treat mental disorders with surgery, despite a limited understanding of their mechanisms, their elusive and varied characteristics and the overall lack of scientific grounding for this method. These operations were performed almost exclusively on women and often resulted in severe mutilation.

Hysteria is a prime example. This term referred to a range of neurotic disorders that mostly affected women, including melancholic mood disorders and depressive dispositions, often entailing somatic symptoms and hypochondria. The concept of hysteria dates back to antiquity, when it was thought to stem from a dysfunctional uterus (the term itself derives from *hysterika*, the Ancient Greek for uterus). The history of hysteria since then is extraordinary, and there are a number of episodes that merit particular attention.

In the eighteenth century, Thomas Willis, the founder of neurology, was particularly fascinated by hysteria. His work paved the way for the Scottish doctor George Cheyne, who had particular success treating what he termed the "English malady" both in London and in Bath. Cheyne used numerous medicines, including "neurotonics" such as iron, strychnine, the bark from a Chinese tree, arsenic and calomel (mercury chloride). He also used opioids (laudanum), emetics, diuretics, laxatives, bloodletting and even the hot springs at Bath.

As surgical techniques and technology progressed, more invasive approaches were adopted. At the height of the Victorian era, for example, the well-known and influential London physician Isaac Baker

Brown performed numerous clitoridectomies, presenting the practice as an effective treatment for various female nervous disorders. His work was widely criticised, both for its ineffectiveness and its futile brutality. Before long, Brown's career collapsed and the practice was abandoned (Sheehan 1981).

In the second half of the nineteenth century it was particularly common for US doctors to use invasive surgical procedures to treat nervous disorders in women. Robert Battey invented the "normal ovariotomy", which involved the surgical removal of healthy ovaries to induce artificial menopause. There was a particularly dramatic case involving a large number of psychiatric patients, many of whom suffered from manic depression and other milder mood disorders. They had the misfortune of being treated at the Trenton State Hospital (New Jersey), which, at the beginning of the twentieth century, was headed by Dr. Henry Cotton. It was his theory that all mental disorders were caused by localised infections and would respond to the surgical removal of the affected organ. He carried out numerous surgical operations on his patients, including explorative laparotomies, the extraction of all the teeth (exodontia), the removal of tonsils, ovaries, bladders, stomachs, spleens, cervixes and colons. There were extremely high levels of intra- and postoperative mortality, and many patients suffered severe mutilation in Dr. Cotton's futile attempts to treat mental disorders. These practices continued for decades until the scandal finally broke and there was a public enquiry into Dr. Cotton's methods. In the event, Dr. Cotton was unable to defend himself because of his own serious psychiatric conditions (Scull 2005).

Despite their ineffectiveness and high operative mortality rates, surgical methods also flourished in Europe because doctors continued to boast of their merits. It would take several decades and many more unnecessarily mutilated women before this approach was finally abandoned (Shorter 1993).

Non-invasive practices were also popular in the Victorian period: one notable example was the "pelvic massage", a euphemism for the masturbation of patients by doctors. In 1880, Joseph Mortimer Granville patented the first electromechanical vibrator, which achieved the same result but with considerably less fatigue for the therapists

(Maines 1999). The use of vibrators has become much more widespread over the years, and Granville's story provides the plot for Tanya Wexler's interesting 2011 film *Hysteria*. The film is grounded in historical fact and shows other medical practices typical of the time, such as bloodletting and electrotherapy.

Other key figures in the history of hysteria include Charcot in Paris, and later Freud in Vienna. The concept of hysteria began to wane at the beginning of the twentieth century (Micale 1993, 2000), however, and was replaced with new nervous disorders (Scull 2009; Shorter 1993; Stepansky 1999; Tasca et al. 2012).

Sigmund Freud had a complex and interesting involvement in the treatment of nervous disorders at the start of his career. It came about in part because of his interest in cocaine. This alkaloid, purified from coca leaves, first became available as a pharmaceutical novelty at the end of the nineteenth century. Around this time, Freud became close friends with the Berlin otolaryngologist Wilhelm Fliess. Fliess was a man of many interests, and he had recently become fascinated by biorhythms, which led to his theory on "nasal reflex neurosis". The theory, published in 1892, proposed a connection between the nose and the genital organs. Fliess believed he had found a link between them because of a number of neurological and psychological symptoms, which he had treated surgically.

On occasion, Freud sent his patients to Fliess for nasal surgery, specifically for the cocainisation of the nasal mucosa (Shorter 1993). A particularly dramatic case was that of Emma Eckstein, a young patient of Freud's, suffering from what was diagnosed as pre-menstrual depression. Freud referred her to Fliess for nasal surgery. When she returned to Vienna after the surgery, her condition worsened steadily. Concerned for his patient, Freud approached a Viennese colleague about the matter. He examined Eckstein and found the cause of her deterioration: a long piece of gauze had been left in the surgical wound. He removed it and Eckstein recovered, but she was left disfigured. She maintained a good relationship with Freud, however, and went on to become a psychoanalyst herself. Freud and Fliess's relationship, on the other hand, ended abruptly due to a mutual misunderstanding (Zucher and Wiegand 1988). Needless to say, Fliess's nasal surgery did not catch on and was soon abandoned.

Fliess used cocaine as a local anaesthetic for nasal surgery, but Freud's involvement with cocaine was substantially more complex. Cocaine was studied much later than most of the other active ingredients from medicinal plants, largely because European researchers struggled to track down samples of the plant *Erythroxylon coca*, from which cocaine was extracted. Cocaine was eventually purified in 1859, and many researchers soon devoted themselves to studying its unique properties—the Italian doctor Paolo Mantegazza and the young Viennese neurologist Sigmund Freud in particular. Freud described it enthusiastically as "a magical drug" in the 1884 article 'Über coca' (Bernfeld 1953). He wrote that cocaine use caused lasting and natural euphoria, alleviated fatigue, hunger and drowsiness, and also fortified intellectual capacity, without resulting in tiredness or depression. It could also be used, he suggested, as a stimulant in war and during trips and climbs. Most importantly, he proposed that it could be used in psychiatry to treat melancholia and neurasthenia. He went on to list other uses, such as treating stomach illnesses, cachexia, typhoid fever, phthisis, syphilis, mercurialism, asthma, alcoholism, morphine addiction and as an aphrodisiac. He also spared a few words for its anaesthetic applications (Bernfeld 1953; Shaffer 1984).

Initial enthusiasm aside, the actual properties of cocaine were quickly recognised. Another researcher, the ophthalmologist Koller, demonstrated that it was an effective local anaesthetic in ophthalmology. This paved the way for its use by other specialists such as dentists. It also laid the foundations for the development of new local anaesthetics free from psychotropic actions (Markel 2011a).

Before long, however, cocaine was found to be seriously addictive and it was soon recognised as a dangerous substance (Musto 1968). Initial attempts to treat opiate addiction with cocaine proved catastrophic, as demonstrated by the dramatic case of Ernst von Fleischl-Marxow. A well-known young Austrian physiologist, he was celebrated for his brilliant studies on the electrical activity of nerves and the nerve structures of the brain. He had been in extreme pain for some time because of a neuroma he developed after the amputation of his thumb. It was treated with analgesic morphine and heroin, a new and even more potent semi-synthetic opiate, and he subsequently developed a serious opiate addiction.

Freud, a close friend of Fleischl-Marxow, procured him cocaine to treat his morphinomania. The situation deteriorated dramatically and Fleischl-Marxow quickly became addicted to cocaine as well as morphine. Ravaged by addiction and pain, he committed suicide at only 45 years of age. Fleischl-Marxow was not the only victim of the addiction: the American surgeon Halsted, who had made outstanding contributions to surgery, suffered from morphinomania. He also tried cocaine to counteract his morphine dependence, only to spend the rest of his life battling the twin addiction of morphine and cocaine (Markel 2011b; Stepansky 1999).

Ernest Jones's official biography ignores Freud's awkward relationship with cocaine, which he initially endorsed enthusiastically as a new elixir to treat a huge variety conditions. He also omits Freud's failure to realise the dangers of cocaine and substance abuse (Karch 1999; Markel 2011b) and to identify its usefulness as a local anaesthetic (Borch-Jacobsen and Shamdasani 2011; Markel 2011a). Despite Freud's endorsement of cocaine and his troubling connection to Fliess, however, he is still remembered as the father of psychoanalysis and of the "talking cure", which was used to treat mental disorders well before the development of pharmacotherapy (Belofsky 2013).

The years following the end of the Second World War saw the identification of the brain's biochemical mechanisms and neurotransmitters, and the development of whole new families of psychiatric drugs that would revolutionise medicine and the treatment of mental disorders. These changes would have a profound effect on psychiatry too, driving the rise of biological psychiatry and the decline of the psychodynamic approach. In the following chapter, I'll examine exactly how this came about.

Notes

1. An official document published by each state, which lists the drugs to prescribe for treating diseases.
2. Liquid confection thought capable of healing all diseases.

References

Abraham, H. D., Aldridge, A. M., & Gogia, P. (1996). The psychopharmacology of hallucinogens. *Neuropsychopharmacology, 14*(285), 285–298.

Basford, J. R. (2001). A historical perspective of the popular use of electric and magnetic therapy. *Archives of Physical Medicine and Rehabilitation, 82,* 1261–1269.

Belofsky, N. (2013). *Strange medicine: A shocking history of real medical practices through the ages.* London: Perigee Book.

Bernfeld, S. (1953). Freud's studies on cocaine, 1884–1887. *Journal of American Psychoanalytic Association, 1*(4), 581–613.

Bethard, W. (2004). *Lotions, potions and deadly elixirs.* Washington: Taylor Trade Publishing.

Booth, C. (2005). The rod of Aesculapios: John Haygarth (1740–1827) and Perkins' metallic tractors. *Journal of Medical Biography, 13*(3), 155–161.

Borch-Jacobsen, M., & Shamdasani, S. (2011). *The freud files: An inquiry into the history of psychoanalysis.* Cambridge: Cambridge University Press.

Crocq, M. A. (2007). Historical and cultural aspects of man's relationship with addictive drugs. *Dialogues in Clinical Neuroscience, 9*(4), 355–361.

Forrest, D. (2002). Mesmer. *International Journal of Clinical and Experimental Hypnosis, 50*(4), 295–308.

Gilman, S. L. (2008). Electrotherapy and mental illness: Then and now. *History of Psychiatry, 19*(3), 339–357.

Haygarth, J. (1800). *Of the imagination, as a cause and as a cure of disorders of the body: Exemplified by fictitious tractors, and epidemical convulsions,* London, Bath. Accessed March 20, 2015, from http://www.jameslindlibrary.org/haygarth-j-1800/.

Karch, S. B. (1999). Cocaine: History, use, abuse. *Journal of the Royal Society of Medicine, 92*(8), 393–397.

Kihlstrom, J. F. (2002). Mesmer, the Franklin commission, and hypnosis: A counterfactual essay. *International Journal of Clinical and Experimental Hypnosis, 50*(4), 407–419.

Maines, R. P. (1999). *The technology of orgasm: "Hysteria," the vibrator, and women's sexual satisfaction.* Baltimore: The Johns Hopkins University Press.

Markel, H. (2011a). Über coca: Sigmund Freud, Carl Koller, and cocaine. *The Journal of the American Medical Association, 305*(13), 1360–1361.

Markel, H. (2011b). *An anatomy of addiction: Sigmund Freud, William Halsted, and the miracle drug cocaine.* New York: Pantheon Books.

Matossian, M. K. (1982). Ergot and the Salem witchcraft affair. *American Scientist, 70*(4), 355–357.

Meggs, W. J. (2009). Epidemics of mold poisoning past and present. *Toxicology and Industrial Health, 25*(9–10), 571–576.

Micale, M. S. (1993). On the "disappearance" of hysteria: A study in the clinical deconstruction of a diagnosis. *Isis, 84*(3), 496–526.

Micale, M. S. (2000). The decline of hysteria. *Harvard Mental Health Letters, 17*(1), 4–6.

Musto, D. F. (1968). A study in cocaine: Sherlock Holmes and Sigmund Freud. *The Journal of American Medical Association, 204*(1), 125–130.

Norton, S. (2006). The pharmacology of mithridatum: A 2000-year-old remedy. *Molecular Interventions, 6*(2), 60–66.

Schwalb, J. M., & Hamani, C. (2008). The history and future of deep brain stimulation. *Neurotherapeutics, 5*(1), 3–13.

Scull, E. (2005). *Madhouse: A tragic tale of megalomania and modern medicine.* New Haven: Yale University Press.

Scull, A., & Schulkin, Y. (2009). Psychobiology, psychiatry, and psychoanalysis: The intersecting careers of Adolf Meyer, Phyllis Greenacre, and Curt Richter. *Journal of Medical History, 53*(1), 5–36.

Shaffer, H. (1984). Uber coca: Freud's cocaine discoveries. *Journal of Substance Abuse Treatment, 1*(3), 205–207.

Sheehan, E. (1981). Victorian clitoridectomy: Isaac Baker Brown and his harmless operative procedure. *Medical Anthropology Newsletter, 12*(4), 9–15.

Shorter, E. (1993). *From paralysis to fatigue: A history of psychosomatic illness in the modern era.* New York: The Free Press.

Shorter, E. (2011). A brief history of placebos and clinical trials in psychiatry. *Canadian Journal of Psychiatry, 56*(4), 193–197.

Shorter, E. (2013). Psychiatry and fads: Why is this field different from all other fields? *Canadian Journal of Psychiatry, 58*(10), 555–559.

Shorter, E., & Healy, D. (2007). *Shock therapy: A history of electroconvulsive treatment in mental illness.* Piscataway: Rutgers University Press.

Spanos, N. P., & Gottlieb, J. (1976). Ergotism and the Salem village witch trials. *Science, 194*(4272), 1390–1394.

Stepansky, P. E. (1999). *Freud, surgery, and the surgeons.* Hillsdale: The Analytic Press.

Tasca, C., Rapetti, M., Carta, M. C., & Fadda, B. (2012). Women and hysteria in the history of mental health. *Clinical Practice & Epidemiology in Mental Health, 8,* 110–119.

Weatherall, M. (1990). *In search of a cure: A history of pharmaceutical discovery.* Oxford: Oxford University Press.

Zuardi, A. W. (2006). History of cannabis as a medicine: A review. *Revista Brasileira de Psiquiatria, 28*(2), 153–157.

Zucher, A., & Wiegand, D. (1988). Freud, fliess, and the nasogenital reflex: Did a look into the nose let us see the mind? In *Otolaryngology Head and Neck Surgery, 98*(4), 319–322.

6

The Rise of Effective Treatments

Medicine is still all about treating populations, not people—one-size-fits all treatments and diagnoses.
Eric Topol

The discovery of the therapeutic effects of medicinal plants gave modern medical therapy a significant boost. In 1747, James Lind demonstrated how the consumption of citrus fruits could prevent scurvy, the terrible vitamin deficiency that struck sailors during long voyages at sea. At the beginning of the seventeenth century, European colonists also discovered that the Peruvian, Bolivian and Ecuadorean people used the bark of a tree to treat malaria. This gave rise to a legend about the bark being used to cure the viceroy of Peru's wife, the Countess of Chinchon. Before long, the bark was known as "Cincona" by the Jesuits, who soon introduced it to Europe, and in 1785 the English physician William Withering showed that the leaves of the poisonous plant digitalis could be used to treat both heart failure and the edema caused by it.

In these early effective treatments, we can actually see the beginnings of modern pharmacotherapy. Soon scientists would begin to identify the active ingredients that made these treatments effective: vitamin C,

© The Author(s) 2017
T. Giraldi, *Unhappiness, Sadness and 'Depression'*,
DOI 10.1007/978-3-319-57657-2_6

quinine, digoxin and digitoxin in the examples above, all of which are still used today. Thanks to advances in the natural sciences, more and more therapeutic breakthroughs soon followed. Botanists discovered new pharmaceutical herbs, and chemists isolated and purified their active ingredients so well-defined molecular forms of them could be prescribed in precise doses (Weatherall 1990).

To start with, new and powerful active ingredients were prepared in forms that were of little practical use, such as drops diluted in water, or powder in swallowable cachets. But pharmaceutical techniques improved greatly in 1894 when Henry Wellcome and his colleague and partner Silas Burroughs invented and patented the "tabloid" tablet, which guaranteed a standard dosage. Wellcome amassed a huge fortune and created a foundation that still supports biomedical research in the UK today. He was also a passionate collector, and his medical library and the many other items he accumulated went on to form a significant part of the London Science Museum's History of Medicine collection. Among the items in the collection is an example of his tabloid, which contained the active ingredients iron, arsenic and digitalis. It's a mixture that would be seen as eccentric and dangerous today because of the inclusion of arsenic, which was used as a tonic (Osborne 1910) but was later abandoned because of its toxic and carcinogenic effects.

These powerful new active ingredients could be used to treat numerous diseases, and even helped with the investigation of human physiology and pathology. It's interesting to note that, historically, new therapeutic methods were almost always identified before the mechanisms of the diseases and medicines in question were fully understood.

The work of biologists and chemists in isolating and identifying natural active ingredients added glycosides, vitamins, hormones and antibiotics to the already known alkaloids. Before long, pharmaceutical chemists were also able to produce synthetic chemicals in their laboratories that could be used effectively in medicine. While investigating the "magic bullet" to combat *Treponema*—which causes syphilis—Paul Ehrlich (1854–1915) synthesised an extensive series of compounds called arsenobenzenes. After producing 605 ineffective derivatives, he eventually found an active one, salvarsan, which paved the way for chemotherapy. In 1908, he and Ilya Ilyich Mechnikov were awarded the Nobel Prize for their work. Extraordinary developments like this in the fields of bacteriology and the study of infectious diseases were to completely revolutionise our understanding of health and disease (Weatherall 1990).

As the pharmaceutical industry grew and progressed, it became more important than ever to develop effective methods for testing the safety and efficacy of new medicines. It was becoming increasingly apparent that the limited objectivity of individual prescribers made it difficult to determine the therapeutic effectiveness and patient tolerance of new medicines. This also hindered attempts to examine the placebo effect (Shorter 2011).

While the medical world was bolstered by a growing number of new powerful and efficient medicines, the therapeutic tools available to nineteenth- and twentieth-century psychiatrists were still decidedly limited. Mithridatum (theriaca) was still in use, as was opium in the form of tincture (laudanum) and mandrake (containing scopolamine). In the mid-nineteenth century many inorganic salts were also in use, such as potassium bromide (a sedative and anticonvulsant), paraldehyde (an anticonvulsant, sedative and hypnotic) and chloral hydrate (a hypnotic). Physical treatments such as hydrotherapy were often used alongside pharmacotherapy.

Modern medicinal substances, created through the synthesis of pharmaceutical chemicals, followed before long. Barbiturates, the first of which was barbital (veronal: a sedative and hypnotic), were introduced in 1903, and this was followed by benzedrine (amphetamine: a psychomotor stimulant) in 1937 (Weatherall 1990). At the same time, however, invasive and debilitating surgical interventions were still being carried out on women in the name of psychiatry. Interventions included mutilating operations on the female sexual organs, dental extractions, colectomies and leucotomies (lobotomies). Malariotherapy (the induction of malaria to cause a fever) was also used to treat syphilis. Endocrine treatments with thyroid and ovarian preparations were also carried out, by Wagner-Jauregg, for example.

There was even the practice of inducing seizures with insulin coma therapy, metrazol (cardiazol) therapy and electric shocks (electroconvulsive therapy). Seen through modern eyes, these treatments seem not only invasive and brutal but also ineffective and lacking in scientific justification. They also often caused irreversible harm to patients. Even though Nobel Prizes were awarded in 1927 to Wagner-Jauregg and in 1949 to Antonio Egas Moniz, their methods are now wholly disregarded (Shorter 1997).

Electroconvulsive therapy (ECT) is still sometimes used for patients suffering from severe depression, but it is falling out of favour. In the past it was also prescribed for those suffering from light or mild mood disorders, and today it is a controversial treatment because of questions about its efficacy and its severe side effects (Jenkusky and Steven 1992; Read and Bentall 2010).

Psychiatric treatment, therefore, was in a fairly dire state in the early twentieth century. This changed dramatically, however, after the Second World War. Pharmacotherapy had hitherto been restricted to a number of sedatives (bromides, paraldehyde, chloral hydrate, barbiturates) and some psychostimulants (amphetamine) (Moncrieff 1999, 2002), and knowledge about the mechanisms of the nervous system was also limited. The discovery of neurotransmission changed all this, however, and accelerated our understanding of the nervous system. We learned that the nervous system was based on the exchange of electrical messages between cells (neurones) through chemical messengers (neurotransmitters). New transmitters were soon discovered, such as dopamine serotonin and both excitatory and inhibitory amino acids. These were added to the transmitters discovered in the peripheral and vegetative nervous system (such as acetylcholine and norepinephrine).

Whole new families of drugs were also accidentally discovered in this period. These drugs, including sedative and anxiolytic benzodiazepines, antipsychotics, antimanic drugs and antidepressants, would soon revolutionise the practice of psychiatry. Studying their properties and mechanisms also led to a deeper understanding of the mechanisms of the brain itself (Brunton et al. 2005; Carlsson 1999; Healy 2002).

It became possible to treat depression effectively in the 1950s, largely because of the antidepressant effects of two new compounds: imipramine and iproniazid They became the heads of two families of drugs: tricyclic antidepressants (TCAs) and monoamine oxidase inhibitors (MAOIs). The interesting story of these two substances can shed light on other developments in psychopharmacology, and so bears further consideration (Moncrieff 2008). A thorough and extensive history of antidepressants can be found in David Healy's book *The Antidepressant Era* (Healy 1997).

The antidepressant effect of imipramine was discovered through the study of a group of organic chemical compounds called phenothiazines These compounds are characterised by a three-ring, six-atom structure in which the central ring contains a sulphur and a nitrogen atom (hence the name pheno-thia-zine). They also have substituents on the atoms that constitute the rings. The French anaesthesiologist Henri Laborit was interested in treatments that mitigated the discomfort experienced during anaesthesia, and was studying the association of anaesthetics with antihistamines. During his study, he used an antihistamine with a phenothiazine structure: promethazine (which is still used as an antihistamine and sedative today).

He noted that, in the patients he treated with it, the sedative effects characteristic of antihistamines were accompanied by a specific loss of interest and responsiveness to environmental stimuli. This led him to wonder whether phenothiazine treatment could help psychotic patients who suffered from an excess of activity and a distortion of their mental functions. Pharmaceutical advances meant that the chemists of the time could quickly synthesise promethazine analogues. Psychiatrists working with Laborit then quickly assessed their clinical properties, and one of these new phenoziathines, chlorpromazine was soon found to be an effective treatment for schizophrenia.

Henri Laborit's later research into psychopharmacology and the functioning of the brain warrants further discussion, but unfortunately that is beyond the remit of this work. He wrote numerous articles and books,[1] and inspired (and also appeared in) Alain Resnais's 1980 film *Mon Oncle d'Amerique*, which offers an unusual depiction of the dawn of psychopharmacology. Such was the importance of his studies that in 1957 he was awarded the prestigious Albert Lasker Award for Clinical Medical Research.

Research that had initially taken place without the support of the pharmaceutical industry thus led to the identification of a revolutionary treatment for some of the symptoms of schizophrenia. Chlorpromazine was quickly followed by a series of new antipsychotic drugs, which would have a profound impact on psychiatric practice, the organisation of psychiatric hospitals and the lives of many schizophrenia sufferers (Preskorn 2010).

Each new medicinal compound, for all its innovation, creates demand for new derivatives that are more active and better tolerated. It is unsurprising, therefore, that this was the case with antipsychotic tricyclic phenothiazines The pharmaceutical company Geigy was interested in the nascent development of antipsychotics and became involved in the study of the relationship between the structure and the effects of tricyclic phenothiazines. This eventually led to the synthesis of the molecule imipramine Structurally it was very close to chlorpromazine the only difference was two carbon atoms instead of a sulphur atom in the compound's central ring.

The new derivative did not produce satisfactory results in schizophrenic patients. Its limited sedative action compared to chlorpromazine, however, convinced the Swiss psychiatrist Roland Kuhn to examine its effects on a group of 40 depressed patients. Its impact was immediate and so marked that after treating just three patients, Kuhn and the doctors and nurses at Geigy had no doubt about the effectiveness of the new treatment. Over the next 3 years the number of patients treated rose to over 500, and it seemed clear that the drug was an efficient antidepressant.

Patients with depression (which was then defined as vital, endogenous or melancholic depression) suffered from retarded thought and action, loss of interest, sleep and appetite disturbances and fixed ideas of helplessness, guilt and desperation. Patients treated with imipramine however, showed increased vivacity and appetite, improved social interactions and a recovery of interest. Their sleep was normalised and patients awoke reporting that they felt positively refreshed, unlike those whose sleep was induced with hypnotic drugs. These improvements often started to appear in the first few days of treatment, and then increased for 3 or 4 weeks.

Kuhn observed that the therapeutic effects of imipramine were symptomatic, and decided that the treatment should be extended. He identified the optimal dose and showed that the treatment could be continued, with tolerable adverse effects for prolonged periods of up to a few years. He also noted the adverse side effects, which were similar to those of antipsychotic phenothiazines dry mouth, copious sweating, constipation, low blood pressure and possible confusion in those suffering from concomitant mental problems. Patients treated with imipramine did not suffer from movement disorders[2] (dyskinesia), however, which was the most significant side effect of antipsychotics (Healy 1997).

Something else that Kuhn observed was that patients often reported (and their relatives confirmed this) that they had not felt this good in a long time. This seems to prefigure the claims made almost 30 years later by advocates and defenders of a new class of antidepressants: selective serotonin reuptake inhibitors (SSRIs), which are examined further below. There were those who claimed that depressed and non-depressed subjects were feeling "better than well", creating the prospect of cosmetic psychopharmacology (Kramer 1997).

This took place a few years after Kuhn's initial observations, when imipramine was becoming more widespread and other researchers were studying its effects. Nathan Kline from the USA is a standout example who reappears later in relation to another family of antidepressants: MAOIs. He is known both for his studies of antidepressants and for the controversy surrounding the discovery of imipramine. Kuhn, however, is generally credited with the initial discovery of the specific antidepressant properties of imipramine, if not its chemical structure.

Despite the effectiveness of the new pharmacotherapeutic treatment for depression, Geigy, the pharmaceutical company involved in its development, doubted there was space for antidepressants in the pharmaceutical market. As a result, they developed and disseminated it slowly to begin with. However, two key events changed their mind. Robert Boehringer, whose family was a major shareholder in the European pharmaceutical company Boehringer Ingelheim, was also a major shareholder in Geigy. When he learned of the effectiveness of imipramine he asked for a sample for one of his relatives who was suffering from depression. They recovered after just a few days of treatment. Unsurprisingly, Boehringer then exerted all his influence to support the industrial development of antidepressants (Fangmann et al. 2008).

The second event was the birth of a new family of antidepressants: MAOIs. This happened, somewhat serendipitously,[3] because of the careful observation of an antituberculosis drug, which led researchers to identify its antidepressant qualities. They then traced this to a group of enzymes.

Monoamine oxidases (MAO) are enzymes that catalyse the oxidative deamination of the neurotransmitters norepinephrine dopamine and serotonin (Slotkin 1999).[4] Our knowledge of this enzyme intersects with the history of the use of hydrazine, a compound with a simple molecular structure that has been known since 1912, and which was used during the Second World War as fuel for the German V1 and V2 rockets. There was a considerable amount of hydrazine left in circulation at the end of the War, and this led the chemical companies who acquired it towards the production of new compounds, including pharmaceutical products. When isoniazid and later iproniazid were synthesised at the beginning of the 1950s, it was found that they could be used in association with the new antibiotic streptomycin to treat tuberculosis (Mitchison and Davies 2012). It was the first effective cure for this widespread disease, and its discovery was one of the great medical achievements of the first half of the twentieth century.

But it was found that iproniazid did not just help to heal tuberculous lesions; it was also an inhibitor of monoamine oxidases and had positive mental side effects. In the Seaview Hospital sanatorium in New York, where black women were hospitalised, doctors observed a marked improvement in mood and found patients dancing in the wards and asking to be discharged, even if they still had tuberculous lesions. These curious side effects found their way into the newspapers of the time too. American and European clinicians became more and more interested in iproniazid, and began to study the psychiatric effects of the compound.

They found that the dosage was critical: high doses administered over prolonged periods could even, they discovered, cause psychotic episodes. However, it appeared clear that, overall, iproniazid increased the vitality of depressed patients (and also caused sharp weight gain). The antidepressant effects of imipramine contrasted with those of amphetamine Amphetamine was administered to depressed patients in the expectation that it would revitalise them, but despite its psychostimulant effect it proved ineffective as an antidepressant and caused a marked loss of appetite and weight. It was eventually abandoned as a treatment for depression (Healy 1997).

MAOIs were developed primarily in the USA, in no small part because of the brilliant psychiatrist Nathan Kline. The pharmaceutical company Roche was also instrumental, despite doubting the market for the new antidepressant. Kline in particular deserves further attention because of his huge role in the development of psychopharmacology and in twentieth-century American psychiatry more generally. Kline is the only researcher to have twice received the Albert Lasker Award for Clinical Medical Research, which is seen as the Nobel Prize of American medicine. He was awarded it in 1957 for his studies of reserpine, and again in 1964 for his work on iproniazid.

In 1952, the alkaloid reserpine was isolated from the plant *Rauwolfia serpentina*, which is used in traditional Indian medicine to treat mental disorders, fever and poisonous snake bites (Stitzel 1976). Reserpine acts on the cardiovascular system and was used as an antihypertensive drug. Patients treated with it became significantly sedated, which led to research into its psychiatric applications. It proved to be an effective treatment for psychotic symptoms in schizophrenic patients, and briefly preceded phenothiazines and butyrophenones as an antipsychotic. When they appeared, however, it was quickly abandoned because of its selectivity and its severe side effects, including movement disorders (dyskinesia) similar to those caused by phenothiazines (Preskorn 2007).

Its complex chemical structure also made it difficult to modify its molecules and thereby study its structure-activity relationships and enhance its safety and effectiveness. This was comparatively easy with synthetic molecules because of their simpler chemical structure, and the process was carried out successfully with phenothiazines, butyrophenones and later with second-generation and atypical drugs (Preskorn 2007).

Because of its effects on psychotic patients, reserpine was designated a tranquiliser, later modified to a "greater tranquiliser" to distinguish it from a new family of drugs "minor tranquilisers". The first in this group was meprobamate, but this was quickly followed by benzodiazepines such as librium and valium, which had selective anxiolytic effects. Minor tranquilisers would soon be widely prescribed by general practitioners, even for non-psychiatric purposes. Their anxiolytic effects, together with the muscle relaxation they caused, meant many started to use them to alleviate everyday tensions and to help them adapt to more minor life events, without the negative image attached to psychiatric drugs. Benzodiazepines were safe in the event of an overdose, unlike barbiturates, which were a frequent cause of acute intoxication and could even be used with suicidal intent. Barbiturate and benzodiazepine dependency became a serious problem (Tone 2009), but I will not go into this in detail here. Suffice it to say that the production and widespread use of barbiturates and benzodiazepines slowed down the development of antidepressants and diverted the interest of pharmaceutical companies, who saw them as more attractive and profitable.

They were finally overtaken approximately 30 years later when a new family of antidepressants emerged: SSRIs (Griebel and Holmes 2013; Horwitz 2010). These had limited adverse side effects in comparison to TCAs and MAOIs, which, again, led to their widespread use, often beyond the confines of psychiatric hospitals.

Looking back at the early 1950s, it is interesting to note that, although reserpine was abandoned in psychiatric pharmacotherapy, extensive studies were carried out on its in vivo effects. These helped to lay the foundations for theories that traced mental disorders to changes in neurochemical mechanisms and cerebral neurotransmission. Reserpine was found to be effective at reducing the cerebral concentration of the neurotransmitters serotonin adrenaline, norepinephrine and dopamine Erminio Costa and Silvio Garattini then showed that imipramine antagonised the sedative effect of reserpine, which led to further attempts to identify new compounds with psychotropic effects. The resulting medicines would be widely used in the following decades.

In fact, numerous biochemical pharmacology studies showed that the properties and interactions of reserpine and iproniazid were far more complex than had been first thought (Curzon 1990). Above all, it was observed that reserpine did not just have a sedative effect: it could actually induce real depression by reducing norepinephrine, dopamine and serotonin levels in the cerebral neurones.

The examination of the structure-activity relationships of active molecules synthesised from tricyclic compounds and MAOIs, therefore, made it possible to conceive of effective pharmacotherapeutic treatments for depression. Interest in antidepressants grew dramatically, and pharmaceutical companies soon began to get involved because they saw a market for this new class of drugs (Moncrieff 2008; Preskorn 2010).

MAOIs—in particular phenelzine and tranylcyprominespread quickly, but only for a short time because severe side effects started to emerge. It turned out that the enzyme inhibition was irreversible and had long-term effects: a minority of patients suffered severe toxicity in the liver and peripheral nervous system, and some even had serious hypertensive crises when they ingested certain foods, while others had severe reactions when they were treated for other concomitant disorders. As a result, although several reversible inhibitors and selective inhibitors were later developed, this class of drugs is now used only when there are no other feasible therapeutic alternatives (López-Muñoz et al. 2007).

A different fate lay in store for the derivatives of imipramine and amitriptyline Extensive studies were carried out on their structure-activity relationships, which led to the discovery of the active molecules—active metabolites—responsible for the in vivo effects of the first TCAs (desipramine, nortriptyline), tricyclic compound derivatives with substituents on the rings (clomipramine and new tricyclic derivatives (doxepin, maprotiline) (Fangmann 2008).

The next major breakthrough in the treatment of depression was the development of fluoxetine (Prozac) by Eli Lilly. This new compound was defined as a SSRI because of its action mechanism. Its antidepressant properties were essentially similar to those of TCAs, but, crucially, it had lower toxicity levels and a higher tolerability profile. As a result, fluoxetine was an unprecedented success: it was introduced into the USA in 1988, and by 1992 it was already making over $1 billion a year in prescriptions. By 2000, the number of patients being treated with fluoxetine had risen to an estimated 38 million.

To begin with, Geigy and Roche were reluctant to invest in the development of antidepressants, deeming it an unprofitable area because of the limited number of patients. But the success of fluoxetine hugely expanded the market and soon pharmaceutical companies were jostling for a share of it. In the space of a few years, other molecules from the SSRI family, such as sertraline, paroxetine, fluvoxamine and citalopram, were launched into the market, and soon these were being prescribed and sold by manufacturers alongside fluoxetine Because these drugs were developed as part of market competition strategies rather than in response to unmet medical needs, their characteristics often overlapped, giving rise to the term "me-too" drugs. However, new compounds with different action mechanisms were developed eventually, and these will be examined in due course (Vaswani et al. 2003).

In this chapter we have seen how it became possible to treat depressive mood disorders using antidepressants that work by increasing the concentration of the neurotransmitters norepinephrine and serotonin in the synaptic cleft. Reserpine, on the other hand, reduces the concentration of norepinephrine and serotonin and acts as a sedative and depressogenic (Castrén 2005). Its ability to reduce the level of dopamine also made it effective as an antipsychotic (Baumeister et al. 2003; Roe 1999). These effects are impressive and observation of them has led to the theory that depression is caused by a deficiency of monoamine neurotransmitters (norepinephrine and serotonin) and that this can be corrected with antidepressants (Castrén 2005). It has also led to the theory that schizophrenia is caused by an excess of dopamine, which can be corrected using antipsychotics (Carlsson and Carlsson 2006; Carlton and Monowitz 1984). These theories have played an important part in our understanding of depression and in the proliferation of antidepressants, and I will examine this in detail in the following chapters.

Notes

1. Many of Laborit's books were widely disseminated, including In praise of flight, The inhibition of action and La Vie anterieure.
2. Iatrogenic Parkinsonism: Parkinson's disease including movement disorders (dyskinesia) such as stiffness and tremors, and similar disorders, are caused by prolonged treatment with antipsychotics (iatrogenic damage caused by medical treatment).
3. It was accidentally discovered (Roberts 1989).

4. In reality there are two forms of enzyme: MAO-A and MAO-B, otherwise present in different tissues. The difference between the two shall not be taken into account here.

References

Baumeister, A. A., Hawkins, M. F., & Uzelac, S. M. (2003). The myth of the reserpine-induced depression: Role in the historical development of the monoamine hypothesis. *Journal of the History of Neurosciences, 12*(2), 207–220.

Brunton, L., Lazo, J., & Parker, K. (2005). *Goodman & Gilman's, the pharmacological basis of therapeutics* (11th ed.). New York: McGraw-Hill Medical.

Carlsson, A. (1999). Birth of neuropsychopharmacology–impact on brain research. *Brain Research Bulletin, 50*(5–6), 363.

Carlsson, A., & Carlsson, M. L. (2006). A dopaminergic deficit hypothesis of schizophrenia: The path to discovery. *Dialogues in Clinical Neurosciences, 8*(1), 137–142.

Carlton, P. L., & Monowitz, P. (1984). Dopamine and schizophrenia: An analysis of the theory. *Neuroscience and Biobehavioral Reviews, 8*(1), 137–151.

Castrén, E. (2005). Is mood chemistry? *Nature Reviews Neurosciences, 6*(3), 241–246.

Curzon, G. (1990). How reserpine and chlorpromazine act: The impact of key discoveries on the history of psychopharmacology. *Trends in Pharmacological Sciences, 11*(2), 61–63.

Fangmann, P., Assion, H. J., Juckel, G., et al. (2008). Half a century of antidepressant drugs: On the clinical introduction of monoamine oxidase inhibitors, tricyclics, and tetracyclics. Part II: tricyclics and tetracyclics. *Journal of Clinical Psychopharmacology, 28*(1), 1–4.

Griebel, G., & Holmes, A. (2013). 50 years of hurdles and hope in anxiolytic drug discovery. *Nature Reviews Drug Discovery, 12,* 667–687.

Healy, D. (1997). *The antidepressant era.* Cambridge, MA: Harvard University Press.

Healy, D. (2002). *The creation of psychopharmacology.* Cambridge, MA: Harvard University Press.

Horwitz, A. V. (2010). How an age of anxiety became an age of depression. *The Milbank Quarterly, 88*(1), 112–138.

Jenkusky, M. D., & Steven, M. (1992). Public perceptions of electroconvulsive therapy: A historic review. *Jefferson Journal of Psychiatry, 10*(2), 3.

Kramer, P. D. (1997). *Listening to prozac: A psychiatrist explores antidepressant drugs and the remaking of the self.* New York: Penguin Books.

López-Muñoz, F., Alamo, C., Juckel, G., et al. (2007). Half a century of antidepressant drugs: On the clinical introduction of monoamine oxidase inhibitors, tricyclics, and tetracyclics. Part I: Monoamine oxidase inhibitors. *Journal of Clinical Psychopharmacology, 27*(6), 555–559.

Mitchison, M., & Davies, G. (2012). The chemotherapy of tuberculosis: Past, present and future. *International Journal of Tuberculosis and Lung Diseases, 16*(6), 724–732.

Moncrieff, J. (1999). An investigation into the precedents of modern drug treatment in psychiatry. *History of Psychiatry, 10*(40), 475–490.

Moncrieff, J. (2002, April 26). Drug treatment in modern psychiatry: The history of a delusion. In *Talk given at Critical Psychiatry network conference, Beyond drugs and custody: Renewing mental health practice.*

Moncrieff, J. (2008). The creation of the concept of an antidepressant: An historical analysis. *Social Science and Medicine, 66*(11), 2346–2355.

Osborne, O. T. (1910). *Handbook of therapy* (2nd ed). The Journal of the American Medical Association. Chicago: American Medical Association.

Preskorn, S. H. (2007). The evolution of antipsychotic drug therapy: Reserpine, chlorpromazine, and haloperidol. *Journal of Psychiatric Practice, 13*(4), 253–257.

Preskorn, S. H. (2010). CNS drug development: Part I: The early period of CNS drugs. *Journal of Psychiatric Practice, 16*(5), 334–339.

Read, J., & Bentall, R. (2010). The effectiveness of electroconvulsive therapy: A literature review. *Epidemiologia e Psichiatria Sociale, 19*(4), 333–347.

Roberts, R. M. (1989). *Serendipity: Accidental discoveries in science.* New York: Wiley.

Roe, D. L. (1999). The discovery of dopamine psysiological importance. *Brain Research Bulletin, 50*(5–6), 375–376.

Shorter, E. (1997). *A history of psychiatry: From the era of the asylum to the age of Prozac.* New York: John Wiley.

Shorter, E. (2011). A brief history of placebos and clinical trials in psychiatry. *Canadian Journal of Psychiatry, 56*(4), 193–197.

Slotkin, T. A. (1999). Mary bernheim and the discovery of monoamine oxidase. *Brain Research Bulletin, 50*(6), 373.

Stitzel, R. E. (1976). The biological fate of reserpine. *Pharmacological Reviews, 28*(3), 179–205.

Tone, A. (2009). *The age of anxiety: A history of America's turbulent affair with tranquilizers*. New York: Basic Books.

Vaswani, M., Linda, F. K., & Ramesh, S. (2003). Role of selective serotonin reuptake inhibitors in psychiatric disorders: A comprehensive review. *Progress in Neuro-Psychopharmacology and Biological Psychiatry, 27*(1), 85–102.

Weatherall, M. (1990). *In search of a cure: A history of pharmaceutical discovery*. Oxford: Oxford University Press.

7

Assessing Efficacy

Hurry, hurry, use the new drug before it stops curing.
Armand Trousseau

Health interventions have become more and more sophisticated over the years, and there has been a corresponding growth in the number of molecular entities and medicines used in therapy. The development of pharmacology, pharmacotherapy and the pharmaceutical industry contributed a great deal to the extraordinary medical progress of the twentieth century, but it has not been a straightforward journey.

Historically, the efficiency and safety of drugs was judged almost entirely by the doctors prescribing them. Their judgements were then shared and debated in scientific society and company meetings, and published in official documents, journals and medical reviews. For many new medicines, their effectiveness was so obvious that there was no need to test it with clinical studies. If anything, a greater challenge was overcoming the conservative resistance of the scientific community. It often took a great deal of time and effort to overturn and replace obsolete, redundant approaches and gain recognition for new and more effective ones. In fact, such was the difficulty of gaining acceptance for

© The Author(s) 2017
T. Giraldi, *Unhappiness, Sadness and 'Depression'*,
DOI 10.1007/978-3-319-57657-2_7

new innovations that many inventors ended up testing them on themselves in public to prove their effectiveness. It was a common practice in medical research for experimenters to try out new treatments on themselves before testing them on patients: it was a generous and ethical approach that saw them running the risks instead of their patients.

A dramatic example of this was the use of activated charcoal as a poison antidote, because of its high absorptivity. The properties of activated charcoal had been known since Hippocratic times but were studied extensively in nineteenth-century France. In 1813, the chemist Bertrand went so far as to swallow five grammes of arsenic trioxide in public to show the effects of activated charcoal. It was a dose that would have proved lethal without an effective antidote, but Bertrand survived without any ill effects. Other researchers also struggled to prove the effects of activated charcoal, however, perhaps because of the difficulty of standardising the preparation method. Sceptical members of the Academy of Medicine challenged another chemist, Pierre-Fleurus Touéry, to prove its antidotal properties. In their presence, Touéry swallowed a gramme of strychnine—10 times the lethal dose for humans. When he survived unharmed, the academics were left in no doubt (Altman 1998).

More recently, in the early 1980s, the Australian scholars Barry J. Marshall and Robin Warren were convinced that gastric ulcers were caused by a curious spiral-shaped microbe called *Helicobacter pylori*. Almost a century after it had been confirmed that infectious diseases could be bacterial in origin, the theory that a serious illness was bacterial was still ridiculed by the scientific establishment. Marshall, frustrated that the scientific community would not accept his observations, ingested a culture of these bacteria and fell sick to gastritis instantly, curing himself with antibiotics later. The scientific community was won over and in 2005 he and Warren were awarded the Nobel Prize in Physiology or Medicine for their research on *Helicobacter pylori* and its role in stomach and pylorus ulcers (Nobel Prize in Physiology and Medicine 2005). There are also a number of other, similar cases, where the results were so conclusive that they could not be called into question (Altman 1998).

As new and more effective approaches were adopted, so archaic, harmful and ineffective methods were gradually abandoned, like the widespread practice of bloodletting. Although there was no evidence for the efficacy of this approach, which was based on the Hippocratic theory of humours, it was widespread right up until the end of the nineteenth century. The use of inorganic or organic arsenic compounds is another example: although today we know arsenic only as a toxic substance, it was commonly used as a tonic until the beginning of the twentieth century. The weight gain and rosy complexion it caused were not signs of recovery but actually the result of damage to the capillary blood vessels (Emsley 2005; Jolliffe 1993).

Some archaic practices are still in use today, such as acupuncture, homeopathy, phytotherapy and chiropractic treatment. They fall into the category of complementary alternative medicine (CAM) (Singh and Ernst 2008) and provoke constant debate about their effectiveness, which is generally limited or unproven.

In the past, the lack of health control mechanisms led to the use of often ineffective and unsafe therapeutic methods, and even when they were shown to be useless and potentially dangerous, overturning these practices was still difficult. Some persisted alongside scientific medicine and even became widespread because of the lack of enforced health control mechanisms in certain countries. Charlatanism wilfully exploits the gullible and is even more repugnant because it preys on the fragility of people in times of suffering. In the nineteenth century the market for patent medicines flourished in England, and even more so in the USA. There was an explosion of panaceas and extravagantly named elixirs such as The Choice Drink of Health, The Original Dr. Stoughton's Elixir, Dr. Bateman's Pectoral Drops, British Oil, Dalby's Carminative, and A Famous Cordial Drink … A Secret … Far Beyond any Medicament Yet Known (Griffenhagen and Young 1959). In the USA, such fanciful pills, cordials and other contrivances persisted for many years until the foundation of the Food and Drug Administration (FDA) in the early twentieth century. This crucial regulatory body has a complex and interesting history, which was accurately recounted by Young in 1961 (Young 1990).[1]

Practically every new scientific innovation has been used in some form or other in medicine, despite often poor and limited justifications, only to be abandoned later—often after a dramatic event. A particularly noteworthy example is Marie Curie and Pierre Joliot's discovery of naturally occurring radioactive elements in 1898. It was an instant sensation, and a host of charlatanic fantasy products quickly followed, such as *THO-RADIA, Creme embellissante parce que curative, a base de thorie et de Rhadium selon la formule du Dr. Alfred Curie, Poudre Scientifique THO-RADIA* and the *Brillantine Scientifique de THO-RADIA vaporisable*, created by a doctor of the same surname (Dr. Alfred Curie), who bore no relation to the discoverers of radium.

The case of Radithor was far more serious. It was a radium salts solution marketed by its inventor William J.A. Bailey as a metabolic stimulant, aphrodisiac and cure for various afflictions. Radithor was popular from 1925 to 1930, until a tragic incident involving the industrialist Eben Byers. Byers was fond of the solution and consumed it in large quantities between 1927 and 1930, but it began to take a toll on his health and in 1932 he passed away because of severe radium poisoning. The case went to court and was widely reported in the press: Radithor was banned and its tragic consequences helped to define the role of regulatory bodies in controlling medicines and radioactive substances (Macklis 1993; Macklis et al. 1990).

Another interesting case is Prontosil, a chemotherapeutic sulphonamide developed by Bayer in 1930s Nazi Germany. It was the first treatment for a large number of bacterial infections.[2] It spread quickly not just because of its effectiveness as an antibacterial agent but also because of the fame it gained when it was used to treat the son of the President of the USA, Franklin Delano Roosevelt, who was dying from severe sinusitis complications. Sulphonamides became controversial in 1935, however, when a group of researchers from the Pasteur Institute in Paris showed that their antibacterial effect was the result of a simple and well-known chemical compound[3] which Prontosil was rapidly metabolised into when it entered the body. To the consternation of the Pasteur Institute researchers, Gerhard Domagk, who discovered the first sulfamide drug sulfamidochrysoïdine, called Prontosil, was awarded the Nobel Prize in Physiology or Medicine in (1939). The researchers, who had shown that the action of sulphonamides was not related to the structure of Prontosil, had some recompense when the Nobel Prize in Physiology or Medicine was awarded to Daniel Bovet in 1957. He was awarded it for discovering the effects of curares on neurotransmission in the central and peripheral nervous system (Hager 2006; Nobel Prize in Physiology and Medicine 1957).

The story of sulphonamides does not end here, however: in 1937 they were also involved in a case of mass poisoning in the USA. Without laws controlling the safety of medicine, Elixir Sulfanilamide was marketed as an antibacterial sulphonamide. It contained an inexpensive active metabolite of Prontosil and used large amounts of another inexpensive chemical substance, ethylene glycol, as a solvent. When taken in large doses, however, ethylene glycol proved to be severely toxic. It killed over 100 people before the product could be completely withdrawn (Hager 2006).

Severe poisoning cases like this, as well as the prevalence of charlatanic, ineffective remedies in the USA, led to a crucial development: the passing of laws to limit the use of non-prescription medicines and ensure only safe and effective treatments were marketed. Ensuring the effectiveness of treatments, however, was no simple matter, because of the difficulty of assessing the activity of drugs.

The USA passed an early form of medicine control legislation in 1902, with the Biologics Control Act. This came about after a serious accident involving a contaminated diphtheria serum, which caused the death of 13 children in St. Louis, Missouri. The next step was the 1906 Food and Drug Act, which banned the inter-state transportation of adulterated food or drugs, whose characteristics were not defined or described adequately, and which were not included in the pharmacopcia of the USA.[4] Then in 1927, the Food, Drug, and Insecticide Administration was created, which 3 years later adopted its current name, the Food and Drug Administration.

It soon became clear, however, that these new measures still didn't prevent the trade of various charlatanic treatments, including radioactive preparations and false treatments for serious illnesses such as tuberculosis and diabetes. Public opinion was an important consideration and the public had already been seriously alarmed by the effects of Radithor and Elixir Sulfanilamide. Another key case was the cosmetic mascara Lash Lure, which used a chemical colourant[5] that turned out to be highly toxic. A certain Mrs. Brown and a quick succession of 15 other victims lost their sight in a matter of hours, and one woman even lost her life because of the mascara (deForest Lamb 1936; Wax 1995).

The 1938 Food, Drug, and Cosmetic Act enforced federal checks on the safety of medicines before they went to market, as well as prohibiting false promises about supposedly miraculous clinical properties. Medical prescriptions also became obligatory, and this was written into law in the 1951 Durham-Humphrey Amendment. The FDA thus came to enforce strict rules about the safety of medicinal products, and was also able to withdraw them following initial authorisation. These rules were further refined in the 1962 Kefauver-Harris Amendment, which stipulated that the safety and efficacy of medicines had to be proved, and this legislation remains in place today (Helm 2007).

These developments show there was a growing need to clearly demonstrate the safety and efficacy of new medicines. On the other hand, the rapid and unhindered progress of clinical science in the first half of the twentieth century made it possible to treat morbid conditions with a range of ever-more sophisticated medicines, which became increasingly difficult to test effectively. Evidently, evaluating results based solely on individual clinical observation was inadequate, as shown by the numerous severe cases of poisoning that shook the public, and while many quack remedies were uncovered, there was still the question of whether the positive results of many effective treatments were caused by active ingredients or the placebo effect (Bracken 2013).

The need to objectively demonstrate the effectiveness of treatments was not new. In 1747, in what is considered the first clinical trial, James Lind tested a number of sailors suffering from scurvy with a range of diets and food sources. He showed that only oranges and lemons worked to clear scurvy, which paved the way for the prophylactic use of citrus juice on long oceanic journeys (Lind 1753).

The first *modern* clinical trial, however, was published in 1948 by the *British Medical Journal* and was to do with the use of streptomycin as a new treatment for tuberculosis, one of history's most virulent and dangerous diseases. The achievements of scientific medicine in the first half of the twentieth century allowed us to gain a much greater understanding of the microbiological and pathological mechanisms of tuberculosis, and substantial resources were invested in treating and preventing it, but without significant results (Daniel 2006). After the discovery of penicillin, however, a second antibiotic streptomycin emerged in the

USA in 1944, and this could be used *in vitro* as a bactericide against *Mycobacterium tuberculosis*, the germ responsible for tuberculosis. The initial results on individual patients were encouraging, and when it arrived in Europe in 1946, the British Medical Research Council, under Austin Bradford Hill, organised a study of the drug's effectiveness.

The study used pioneering methods that were later incorporated into the methodology of modern randomised clinical trials (RCTs). 55 patients treated with streptomycin were tested against 52 control patients, and an objective improvement was observed in 31 of the patients treated and 16 of the control patients. There were 12 deaths among those treated and 24 among the control patients (Crofton 2006; Medical Research Council Investigation 1948). The results were validated with statistical analysis, and streptomycin became an essential antituberculosis drug, particularly in conjunction with other active ingredients. The first of these to be proved effective were isoniazid and iproniazid, which have already been mentioned as two of the first antidepressants—discovered in antituberculosis sanatoriums, thanks to their positive effect on the patients' moods.

The methodological principles used in the trial of streptomycin were adopted for clinical trials from then on (Bracken 2013). They include:

- Randomisation—the distribution of the patients in the treatment or control group using mathematically valid principles of randomness
- Double blind—not informing the patients, practitioners or assessors about the status of the patients at the end of the trial, particularly which treatments were given to the different patients
- Control—the rigorous definition of each patient's condition at the start and end of each treatment

Such is the difficulty of assessing the safety and efficacy of new medicines that it is still a matter of much debate today. Nevertheless, there has been solid consensus about the gold standard of assessment since the 1950s: the benchmark for clinical trials is the RCT. The characteristics that validate a clinical trial are clearly outlined in a set of protocols with which investigators have to comply. This is an example of a simple set of protocols:

- The disease which afflicts the subjects to be included (enrolled) in the study should be clearly and objectively defined by characteristics such as nature and severity.
- The demographic (e.g. age, sex, marital status, occupation) and clinical characteristics (e.g. previous illnesses, any other existing illness, and childbearing or menopausal status in the case of women) of the subjects who will be enrolled in the study should be accurately defined, to exclude inhomogeneities on entering the trial which may affect its results.
- The assessment criteria of the expected therapeutic response (outcome) should be precisely defined as per nature and severity.
- Groups of patients, randomly selected with a precise mathematical procedure (randomisation), should undergo the treatment under examination, compared with a reference group treated with a placebo[6] and a possible control group with the best treatment currently available (the "arms" of the treatment trial).
- The treatment should be carried out without the enlisted subjects and the doctors and nurses involved in the treatment and assessment of its efficacy knowing the nature of the preparation administered to each patient (containing the new drug, no active substance for the placebo arm or the possible active drug comparator), leading to the "double blind" condition; the real data of the patients undergoing different treatments under trial can only be analysed at the end of the trial.
  "Informed consent" should be obtained from every patient enrolled in the study.

There is another crucial ethical consideration when carrying out clinical trials: namely that investigators have to obtain informed consent. This is a core part of the ethical standards for all health treatments, and in particular for medical experimentation on humans. These standards were outlined by the Nuremberg trials at the end of the Second World War, which examined the crimes committed by German physicians during the war. They were adopted by international treaties, the most important of which was the World Medical Association's 1954 Declaration of Helsinki, which was followed by a series of amendments and other documents, such as the 1995 *Guidelines for Good Clinical Practice for Trials on Pharmaceutical Products* WHO (1995).

The ethical guidelines for clinical trials were a hugely important breakthrough. Over time, the regulatory authorities of different countries have enforced similar guidelines, ensuring that new drugs can only be introduced into the market after clinical trials. These trials have to be RCTs carried out on individuals who have been properly informed and have explicitly expressed their informed consent. An important consequence of this is that all participants understand that they are taking part in clinical trials in which they could receive experimental drugs, placebos or established treatments.

The aim of all this is to ensure that the effectiveness of treatments is irrefutably established by RCTs. Of course, this is only possible thanks to the generous and altruistic decision of patients to take part. But asking patients to take part in trials where they could receive either a new treatment or a placebo is much more problematic, and this practice is not used in trials for treatments for serious illnesses such as cancer, where it would be unacceptable to withhold effective treatment from patients. Placebos are used in trials for antidepressants, however. This may imply a lack of faith in the effectiveness of new antidepressants, because researchers are only willing to test them against placebos and not against the antidepressants already on the market (Kaptchuk 1998; Timmermans and Berg 2003).

It is worthwhile considering a number of other regulations used to determine whether drugs are safe and effective enough to bring to market (Brody 2012):

- The overall procedure of this clinical trial should be initially authorised by a specific structure, accredited by the national regulatory body, which can take a different shape (ethics committee,   review board, etc.). It should be authorised to consent to (or refuse) the execution of the clinical trial in line with the proposed protocol, if the evidence of the pre-clinical trials on its efficacy and safety are considered sufficient to expose participants to a clinical trial at the risk of scarce clinical action and unexpected adverse effects.

- The organisation of the trial includes different phases. Phase 1, normally using healthy volunteers, determines safe dosages and means of administering them, to be used in the later phases. Phase 2 ascertains whether there is a significant therapeutic response. Phase 3 entails comparison with the treatment already available (or with a placebo).
- If Phase 3 is passed successfully, the new medicine is marketed and Phase 4 begins: post-marketing surveillance. The regulatory body collects all reports on the therapeutic effects and particularly adverse effects that occurred during use in current clinical practice.
- During Phases 1–3 of the trial, for the obvious ethical reason of containing the number of volunteers exposed to the risks of ineffectiveness and the danger inherent in clinical experimentation, the number of participants is limited to the minimum necessary to obtain statistically significant results. After the initial authorisation for marketing, the largest number of patients treated can reveal severe adverse effects caused by the treatment in a relatively infrequent manner and therefore undetectable by the minimum number used in clinical trials. In these cases, the regulatory authority may order the medicine to be withdrawn from the market.

The effectiveness of double-bind, randomised, placebo-controlled trials has led to their use in psychiatry. The very first example was probably a 1954 study into the treatment of manic patients with lithium. It showed the high effectiveness of the treatment (Schou et al. 1954) and as a result lithium is still in widespread use today. At around the same time, however, there was also a curious case involving reserpine, which was then being used as an antihypertensive and antipsychotic (Preskorn 2007). All the pharmacology and medical therapy textbooks of the time reported that patients treated with reserpine often suffered from serious mood disturbances as a side effect. But when a randomised, placebo-controlled trial was conducted into the effects of reserpine on patients suffering from depression and anxiety, it was found that reserpine could have significant antidepressant effects. Reserpine was the subject of one of the first psychiatric studies to use effective modern scientific methods, and it showed the drug had a safe antidepressant action (Davies and Shephers 1955), contradicting the widespread belief that it was a depressogenic (Baumeister 2003).

Using the placebo effect in clinical trials was a major breakthrough in the assessment of the effectiveness of treatments, but more recently the FDA's regulations have drawn increasing criticism because they allow the marketing of new psychiatric drugs that have only been tested against placebos instead of existing drugs. It is even claimed that the scientific integrity of many controlled RCTs has been compromised so they can serve as a marketing tool (Shorter 2011).

After the Second World War, increasingly strict regulations for the assessment, marketing and prescription of medicines paved the way for major advances in basic science and clinical medicine and extraordinary leaps forward in pharmacotherapy. Many new active molecular entities were identified and developed, bringing about a revolution in the treatment of illnesses. These new molecular entities were enormously profitable for the pharmaceutical industry, allowing it to grow on a multinational scale. Each company had at least one drug that brought in a turnover of over a billion dollars a year—the so-called "blockbuster" —along with a spread of "me-too" drugs practically identical to those already marketed by other companies, whose *raison d'être* was to make extra profit in other market sectors (Angell 2004).

During the same period, the development of new medicines gradually shifted from universities and teaching hospitals to pharmaceutical companies and private research bodies and clinics. Soon the marketing costs of new drugs escalated to such an extent that it became impossible for public organisations to compete, pushing their development further and further into the private sphere (Krimsky 2003; Washburn 2005). By the end of the 1990s, the cost of marketing a new drug was estimated to be 800 million dollars, and that figure is still rising today (Adams 2006; Goozner 2004).

This is the current state of affairs for medicinal drugs in general, but now it's time to look more closely at antidepressants.

Notes

1. Detailed information on quackery and fraud in medicine can be found on the website Quackwatch, edited by Dr. Stephen Barrett. The Museum of Questionable Medical Devices (http://www.museumof-quackery.com/) can also be consulted. The collections have been exhibited at the Science Museum of St. Paul, Minnesota since the founder's death in 2010 (Museum of Questionable Medical Devices).
2. Sulphonamides are mainly active against a group of round-shaped bacteria, Gram-positive cocchi, which can be identified in the laboratory using specific staining procedures.
3. Para-amino-benzene-sulphonamide.
4. One curious case is that of Wilhelm Reich, a first-generation psychoanalyst who abandoned Europe and emigrated to the USA in 1939. He developed the concept of orgone energy and orgone accumulators (wooden containers lined with metallic sheets used to cure mental disorders), which he produced and sent, together with books and leaflets, to various patients in different states. The FDA ordered him to stop the inter-state shipment of these materials, judging them to be "adulterated" and not proven to have therapeutic properties. Reich ignored the injunction and was condemned to 2 years in prison, during which he died of a heart attack. In one of the most serious cases of censorship to have occurred in the USA, the court ordered six tonnes of his books to be incinerated (Greenfield 1974).
5. Para-phenylenediamine.
6. The placebo is a pharmaceutical form (tablet, capsule, solution, etc.) identical to the trial one minus the specific active compound under assessment.

References

Adams, C. P., & Brantner, V. V. (2006). Estimating the cost of new drug development: Is it really $802 Million? *Health Affairs, 25*(2), 420–429.
Altman, L. K. (1998). *Who goes first. The story of self-experimentation in medicine*. Berkley: University California Press.

Angell, M. (2004). *The truth about the drug companies. How they deceive us and what to do about it.* New York: Random House.

Baumeister, A. A., Hawkins, M. F., & Uzelac, S. M. (2003). The myth of the reserpine—induced depression: Role in the historical development of the monoamine hypothesis. *Journal of the History of Neurosciences, 12*(2), 207–220.

Bracken, M. B. (2013). *Risk, chance and causation. Investigating the origins and treatment of diseases.* New Haven, CT: Yale University Press.

Brody, T. (2012). *Clinical trials. Study design, endpoints and biomarkers, drug safety, FDA and ICH guidelines.* Amsterdam: Elsevier.

Crofton, J. (2006). The MRC randomized trial of streptomycin and its legacy: A view from the clinical front line. *Journal of Royal Society of Medicine, 99*(10), 531–534.

Daniel, T. M. (2006). Historical review. *The history of tuberculosis, in respiratory medicine, 100*(11), 1862–1870.

Davies, D. L., & Shepherd, M. (1955). Reserpine in the treatment of anxious and depressed patients. *Lancet, 269*(6881), 117–120.

deForest Lamb, R. (1936). *American chamber of horrors: The truth about food and drugs.* New York: Farrar & Rinehart.

Emsley, J. (2005). *The elements of murder.* Oxford: Oxford University Press.

Goozner, M. (2004). *The $800 million pill. The truth behind the cost of new drugs.* Oakland: University of California Press.

Greenfield, J. (1974). *Wilhelm reich vs. the U.S.A.* New York: W.W. Norton & Company Inc.

Griffenhagen, G. B., & Young, J. II. (1959). *Old English patent medicines in America.* Washington: Smithsonian Institution.

Hager, T. (2006). *The demon under the microscope. From battlefield hospitals to Nazi labs, one doctor's heroic search for the world's first miracle drug.* New York: Harmony Books.

Helm, K. A. (2007). Protecting public health from outside the physician's office: A century of FDA regulation from drug safety labeling to off-label drug promotion. *Fordham Intellectual Property, Media & Entertainment Law Journal.* Retrieved May 30, 2016, from http://www.stblaw.com/docs/default-source/Publications/200flspub9537.pdf?sfvrsn=2.

Jolliffe, D. M. (1993). A history of the use of arsenicals in man. *Journal of the Royal Society of Medicine, 86*(5), 287–289.

Kaptchuk, T. J. (1998). Powerful placebo: The dark side of the randomised controlled trial. *Lancet, 351*(9117), 1722–1725.

Krimsky, S. (2003). *Science in the private interest. Has the lure of profits corrupted biomedical research?* Lanham: Rowman & Littlefields Publishers Inc.

Lind, J. (1753). http://inspire.stat.ucla.edu/unit_04/scurvy.pdf. Accessed 10 Mar 2014.

Macklis, R. M. (1993). The great radium scandal. *Scientific American, 269*(2), 94–99.

Macklis, R. M., Bellerive, M. R., & Humm, J. L. (1990). The radiotoxicology of radithor. Analysis of an early case of Iatrogenic poisoning by a radioactive patent medicine. *The Journal of American Medical Association, 264*(5), 619–621.

Medical Research Council Investigation. (1948). Streptomycin treatment of pulmonary tuberculosis. *British Medical Journal, 2*(4582), 769–782.

Nobel Prize in Physiology and Medicine. (1939). http://www.nobelprize.org/nobel_prizes/medicine/laureates/1939/domagk-facts.html. Accessed 13 Mar 2014.

Nobel Prize in Physiology and Medicine. (1957). http://www.nobelprize.org/nobel_prizes/medicine/laureates/1957/bovet-facts.html. Accessed 14 Mar 2014.

Nobel Prize in Physiology and Medicine. (2005). http://www.nobelprize.org/nobel_prizes/medicine/laureates/2005/. Accessed 13 Mar 2014.

Preskorn, S. H. (2007). The evolution of antipsychotic drug therapy: Reserpine, chlorpromazine, and haloperidol. *Journal of Psychiatric Practice, 13*(4), 253–257.

Schou, M., Juel-Nielsen, N., Strömgren, E., et al. (1954). The treatment of manic psychoses by the administration of lithium salts. *Journal of Neurology Neurosurgery and Psychiatry, 17*(4), 250–260.

Shorter, E. (2011). A brief history of placebos and clinical trials in psychiatry. *Canadian Journal of Psychiatry, 56*(4), 193–197.

Singh, S., & Ernst, E. (2008). *Trick or treatment; alternative medicine on trial.* London: Bantam Press.

Timmermans, S., & Berg, M. (2003). *The gold standard: The challenge of evidence-based medicine and standardization in health care.* Philadelphia: Temple University Press.

Washburn, J. (2005). *University, Inc. The corporate corruption of American higher education.* New York: Basic Books.

Wax, P. M. (1995). Elixirs, diluents, and the passage of the 1938 federal. *Food, Drug and Cosmetic Act, in Annals of Internal Medicine, 122*(6), 456–461.

WHO. (1995). World Health Organization. WHO technical report series, no. 850, 1995, Annex 3. Guidelines for good clinical practice (GCP) for trials on pharmaceutical products.

Young, J. H. (1990). *The toadstool millionaires: A social history of patent medicines in America before federal regulation.* In Quackwatch. http://www.quackwatch.com/13Hx/TM/00.html. Accessed 7 Mar 2014.

8

The Effectiveness of Antidepressants Today

Fourth Law: For every expert there is an equal and opposite expert.
Arthur C. Clarke

The effectiveness of monoamine oxidase inhibitors (MAOIS, such as iproniazid and tranylcypromine) and tricyclic derivatives (like imipramine and amitriptyline) for patients with severe forms of depression was evident right from the start. The first antidepressants, however, were essentially limited to the psychiatric sphere, and this was the main reason why the pharmaceutical industry believed there was only a limited number of people who could be treated with this new type of drug. It therefore seemed unlikely to be profitable, which limited pharmaceutical companies' interest in developing new drugs and improving existing ones. This was a serious problem because the soaring costs of pre-clinical and clinical trials meant that private pharmaceutical companies were the only institutions that could afford to develop new drugs.

Two events changed all this. First, the marked effectiveness of new antipsychotic drugs in alleviating the symptoms of schizophrenia encouraged a profound shift in psychiatric practice and created a profitable market for pharmaceuticals. Second, a new family of drugs was

© The Author(s) 2017
T. Giraldi, *Unhappiness, Sadness and 'Depression'*,
DOI 10.1007/978-3-319-57657-2_8

discovered: benzodiazepines (BDZs). They were first described as "minor tranquilisers" to distinguish them from "major tranquilisers". Before long, however, the term "tranquiliser" was dropped and minor tranquilisers came to be described as "anxiolytics", and major tranquilisers were renamed "antipsychotics". Meprobamate, a carbamate derivative, was the first anxiolytic drug and was quickly followed by BDZs such as chlordiazepoxide (librium) and diazepam (valium). These new drugs were destined for widespread use because they could be taken outside the confines of psychiatric hospitals and without psychiatric prescription, through general practice and even self-prescription (Tone 2009).

Unlike the barbiturates that had preceded them, BDZs (colloquially known as "benzos" in the Anglo-Saxon world) were safe drugs, so there was almost no risk that patients would attempt to use them for acute intoxication or suicidal intent. Their specific anxiolytic action was accompanied by muscle relaxation and mild sedation, which made them ideal for mitigating the discomfort and tension of the hyperactive, competitive lifestyle typical of the USA. It was found that BDZs worked by strengthening the inhibitory action of a recently discovered neurotransmitter, γ-aminobutyric acid (GABA). This mechanism was completely different from those of antipsychotics and antidepressants.

In the USA, BDZs were marketed as "useful against the stress of everyday life", which helped to topple the stigma traditionally associated with psychiatric medication, and helped to turn them into blockbuster[1] drugs.[2] The problem of tolerance, and in particular the psychological and physical dependence caused by prolonged use, was scarcely considered in the years immediately following their introduction. But this became a cause of serious concern in later years. Interestingly, this happened around the time when BDZs' patent expired and they became far less profitable. It was also around this time that a second generation of antidepressants appeared, which were better tolerated. These then became great blockbusters too, and were recommended for anxiety disorders that had previously been treated with BDZs, despite their highly distinct mechanisms and the great variety of neurochemical mechanisms associated with anxiety and depression (Tone 2009).

The methodology of clinical trials was refined during this period and the gold standard became double-blind prospective randomised controlled trials (RCTs). The legislation for authorising drugs also pro-gressed in this period, and regulatory bodies were established, such as the Food and Drug Administration (FDA) in the USA, as well as many others in Europe and elsewhere. But new regulations also meant that the cost of developing and having new drugs authorised became so exorbitant that only multinational pharmaceutical companies could afford it. The estimated cost stood at 800 million dollars at the end of the 1990s and surged to 2.6 billion in subsequent years. It should, however, be noted that these estimates were criticised in many quar-ters (Adams 2006, 2010; Goozner 2004; Mullin 2014). The US mar-ket is undoubtedly the largest and also the most important in terms of scientific and industrial development, so this book will focus on how the FDA determines the effectiveness of antidepressants and authorises them for the market. The FDA's work is also of great significance for regulatory bodies in other countries.

In 1977, the FDA published a document entitled *Guidelines for the Clinical Evaluation of Antidepressant Drugs*, which was fully integrated—with no significant changes—into the document *Guidance for Industry*. It sets out in detail the procedures for correctly conducting clinical trials, and subdivides them into Phases 1, 2 and 3. Some of the most important features are detailed in Phase 2; they cover both the selec-tion of subjects and the characterisation of depressive disorders. The *Guidelines* acknowledge that:

> In evaluation of antidepressant drugs, major problems arise from the semantic confusions associated with multiple meanings of the term "depression". … In clinical psychiatry, the two uses that are most per-tinent to drug investigations are depression as a symptom and as a syn-drome. As a symptom, depression may occur in association with other mental, behavioural, and psycho-physiological manifestations in various, and as yet poorly understood, complex combinations.

It is also recognised that:

> **We also do not have normative data for distinguishing between the normal depressive state and the pathologic symptom.**[3]

Some preliminary psychometric studies have been undertaken by Beck, Katz, Zung and others; and research efforts are underway using population survey and epidemiologic techniques to generate such norms.

Although the fundamental distinction between normal and pathological states is rightly mentioned, this detail is lost in the mountain of information about the diagnosis of depression. At the same time, the description of depression and drug evaluation in this document corresponds with the diagnostic criteria established by the American Psychiatric Association's (APA) *Diagnostic and Statistical Manual of Mental Disorders* (DSM):

The most common clinical conditions for which antidepressant drugs are tested are the various depressive syndromes. "Syndrome" refers to the temporal coexistence and covariation of related symptoms and behaviours. Patients with a depressive syndrome usually manifest a depressed mood (as described below) and four or more associated symptoms:

1. Depressed mood characterised by: sadness, feeling low, despondent, hopeless, gloomy.
2. Anhedonia—inability to experience pleasure.
3. Poor appetite or weight loss.
4. Sleep difficulty (insomnia or hypersomnia).
5. Loss of energy, fatigue, lethargy.
6. Agitation.
7. Retardation.
8. Decrease in libido.
9. Loss of interest in work and usual activities.
10. Feelings of self-reproach or guilt.
11. Diminished ability to think or mixed-up thoughts.
12. Thoughts of death/suicide.
13. Feelings of helplessness and hopelessness.
14. Anxiety or tension.
15. Bodily complaints.

Global scales are used to assess the changes observed after treatment, such as psychometric questionnaires like clinical interview schedules

(Hamilton, Levi, Overall, Spitzer, Wittenborn), the Menninger Health-Illness Scale, and patient self-rating scales like those created by Zung and Beck (FDA 1997).

Evidently, assessment depends entirely on the psychometric scale used. Extensive use suggests that the Hamilton Rating Scale for Depression (HRSD) is particularly effective for reflecting the mood disorder symptoms described in the various editions of the DSM, and for detecting any changes caused by antidepressants—particularly first-generation ones. Among the other scales used, the Beck Depression Inventory is especially effective for highlighting cognitive changes. This is hardly surprising as the scale was designed both to identify patients suffering from mood disorders who could be treated with cognitive behavioural psychotherapy, and to determine the effectiveness of the treatment (Healy 1997; Beck 1995; Leucht et al. 2013).

The HRSD is the psychometric scale most widely used for assessing the effectiveness of antidepressants. It was originally made up of 17 items[4] (Hamilton 1960), but this was extended to 21 in later versions (Hamilton 1967), and there are many more versions with varying amounts of changes. The items in the HRSD are graded according to severity, some on a three-point scale (0–2) and others on a five-point scale (0–4), to give an overall score at the end. When psychiatrists give an initial diagnosis of depression, according to the DSM diagnostic criteria, they then conduct a clinical interview using the HRSD to outline the severity of the disorder and the change caused by treatment. The scale's 17 items should now be examined in more detail:

1. Depressed mood (feelings of sadness, hopelessness, helplessness, worthlessness).
2. Guilt.
3. Suicide.
4. Initial insomnia.
5. Middle insomnia.
6. Delayed insomnia.
7. Work and interests.
8. Retardation (ideation, speech, lack of concentration, motor disturbance).

9. Agitation.
10. Anxiety (psychic symptoms).
11. Anxiety (most common somatic symptoms: dry mouth, flatulence, belching, indigestion, diarrhoea, abdominal cramps, palpitations, headaches, hyperventilation, sighing, frequent urination, excessive sweating).
12. Gastro-intestinal symptoms.
13. General somatic symptoms (heavy limbs, back or head, headache or backache, muscular aching, loss of energy and easily tired).
14. Loss of libido.
15. Hypochondriasis.
16. Loss of weight.
17. Loss of insight.

Despite the widespread use of the HRSD and the DSM's major depressive disorder diagnosis, there are still no official or scientific criteria to determine the severity of depression.

As it stands, a score of between 7 and 10 is deemed to reflect the absence of depression, while up to 17 is considered mild depression, 18–24 is moderate, and over 24 is severe. The process of assessing antidepressants at the end of recruitment[5] can account for scores on the threshold of mild or moderate depression. According to the APA, however, the severity of depression is mild if the score is between 8 and 13, moderate between 14 and 18, severe between 19 and 22, and very severe if over 22 (Rush et al. 2000).

The first studies of antidepressants came about after the observation of the effects of iproniazid and imipramine In the years after this, MAOIs were quickly abandoned and tricyclic derivatives were developed. In the 1980s, after a boom in prescriptions, tricyclic derivatives were joined by a new class of second-generation compounds: selective serotonin reuptake inhibitors (SSRIs). New drugs with mixed and atypical mechanisms were also developed. All of these were approved by the FDA using the procedures described above, and by other regulatory bodies using a variety of methods. Almost all the clinical trials carried out used the gold standard of the double-blind randomised, placebo-controlled trial and the effectiveness of treatments was determined by the reduction of patients' HRSD scores.

There are an enormous number of antidepressant studies available: in the US National Library of Medicine—National Institutes of Health database, a search of the keyword "depression" brings up a total of 303,369 works published between 1968 (when there were 2518) and 2012 (17,964 were carried out in that year alone). The search "antide-pressant drug" brings up a total of 122,039 between 1968 (1369) and 2012 (3909). The number of antidepressants marketed after initial observations of imipramine is equally high.

A large part of the study of antidepressants has been dedicated to their action mechanisms, and today antidepressants are generally grouped according to their mechanism and chemical structure. The action mechanisms of antidepressants are particularly important because they relate to the question of whether depressive disorders are caused by a shortage of neurotransmitters such as norepinephrine and serotonin. If this is the case, there is the further question of whether antidepres-sants can effectively correct this deficiency. These are extremely impor-tant matters and they have been the subject of much experimentation and debate. They will be examined in greater detail later on, but for now let's consider how they relate to the antidepressants on the market.

The first thing to observe is that the number of compounds in use at the moment is rather high: the FDA lists 38 overall (FDA 2015). The number of medicines on the market is fairly evenly distributed between the different action mechanisms (although there are some differences between the categorisations of different authors)   (Brunton 2005). There are eight tricyclic antidepressants (TCAs), along with five newer tetracyclic compounds (TeCAs).[6] There are also five MAOIs (RIMA, reversible monoamine inhibitors), with different reversibility properties depending on the two forms of enzyme targeted.[7] Certain TCAs con-tinue to be prescribed for some forms of severe depression, although generally they have been replaced by SSRIs. MAOIs have been practi-cally abandoned because of their pronounced adverse effects although there are now new reversible compounds with greater selectivity. Overall, it seems that they have been abandoned not so much because of safety concerns and limited effectiveness but rather because of the industry's lack of interest (Shulman et al. 2013).

The eight SSRIs are the drugs most commonly prescribed nowadays, and their progenitor fluoxetine (Prozac) has been a major success for the pharmaceutical industry. During the validity of its patent, from 1987 to 2002, Prozac was prescribed to 40 million people and made sales of 22 billion dollars. The American magazine *Fortune* proclaimed it one of "[t]he pharmaceutical products of the century" (Wong et al. 2005), partly because of its greater tolerability, and fluoxetine is now used not just for depressive mood disorders but for a whole array of psychiatric conditions.

In terms of action mechanisms, TCAs inhibit the uptake of both norepinephrine and serotonin the great innovation of SSRIs was that they selectively inhibited the uptake of just serotonin. There are also two selective norepinephrine reuptake inhibitors (NRIs) on the market, and three more recent molecules that, like TCAs, inhibit the uptake of norepinephrine and serotonin (SNRIs) but with less pronounced side effects.

There are also 18 compounds that are defined as "atypical", and these have a range of other mechanisms. Broadly speaking, they antagonise different neurotransmitter brain receptors through serotonin, norepinephrine, dopamine acetylcholineendogenous opioids and excitatory amino acids, one of the drugs that acts as a stimulant for melatonin receptors. There are also other molecules with other properties, as well as numerous new compounds in different phases of pre-clinical and clinical experimentation (Murrough and Charney 2012). The number of antidepressants mentioned here also excludes some that were initially approved and later withdrawn from the market because they were deemed to be toxic (Fung et al. 2001). Including these would make for an extremely long list.

All these antidepressants entered the market through the process described above. In the USA, the FDA authorises medicines after gold-standard clinical trials (RCTs) against placebos have proved they consistently reduce major depressive disorder in patients by at least three points on the HRSD. In the UK, the National Institute for Health and Care Excellence (NICE) also set the threshold at three points, but then removed this guideline (NICE 2004, 2009).

Most published studies use limited patient groups, and their protocols vary significantly and are often not immediately comparable.

A joint review of more studies could lead to greater numerical consistency and a greater understanding of the results: but is this possible considering the varied protocols?

Meta-analysis, a technique that enables the joint analysis of results from a range of studies on the same subject, was one tool developed to answer this question. On the one hand, the most important criteria for critical evaluation are the nature and degree of the effects observed (primary outcome and clinical significance). On the other hand, it must be certain that the results occur in a non-random and repeatable way (statistical significance). As well as trial enrolment, the outcomes are obviously important too—for example: score reduction on a questionnaire, the percentage of patients in which it occurs, the complete disappearance of symptoms, response duration, and progress in comparison with a placebo-controlled group (or possibly the known evolution of the disease).

American epidemiologists consider the first critical approaches to trials to be those developed by Joseph Goldberger at the turn of the nineteenth century, in 1906. His work on pellagra and typhoid fever is not well known today, but it was hugely significant: both illnesses were not well understood at the time (Elmore and Feinstein 1994).

The English epidemiologist Archie Cochrane also made significant contributions to the development of stringent randomised trials. In fact, he helped to lay the foundations for the development of evidence-based medicine, which spurred on meta-analysis and the critical review of controversial clinical problems. His work was also taken up and continued by an excellent group of researchers through the international Cochrane Collaboration (Bracken 2013; Cochrane 2016). Individual articles were published in specialist reviews and the overall amount of reviews, critical reviews and meta-analysis grew, particularly through the Cochrane Collaboration's database.

Irving Kirsch's (1998) meta-analysis, entitled *Listening to Prozac but Hearing Placebo: A Meta-Analysis of Antidepressant Medication* (Kirsch and Sapirstein 1998), caused considerable uproar. It was published in the APA's online magazine, accompanied by a surprisingly long editor's note, in which the editor essentially distanced himself from the article despite agreeing to publish it. Kirsch's work selected 19 published studies, all of which were sufficiently rigorous (RCTs), to be considered in the meta-analysis. The placebo response of control-group patients was consistent across all the studies and correlated strictly with the magnitude of the treatment response. The placebo effect accounted for 75% of the total response of the groups treated with antidepressants, meaning the effects of antidepressant treatment only accounted for 25% of the overall response observed (Kirsch and Sapirstein 1998).

The work was criticised principally for the choice of studies, even though they were chosen for their high standards. There was also the problem that, as well as published results, there were also unpublished results to which Kirsch did not have access. Industry confidentiality meant the pharmaceutical companies that held the patents and sponsored the studies were not obliged to publish or communicate these results to the regulatory body.

To counteract the criticisms of the meta-analysis, the unpublished data had to be included. Kirsch had to resort to the US Freedom of Information Act (FOIA), which grants access to confidential data if it is in the interest of US citizens. As a result, he was able to gain access to the original data from the clinical trials, which concerned six of the seven SSRI antidepressants approved by the FDA between 1987 and 1992. The stated purpose of Kirsch and his colleagues' work was to assess whether the inclusion of the unpublished data would change the results of the first meta-analysis. They also wanted to assess whether the results depended on the severity of the mood disorder. When the HRSD score of each group of patients was related to the severity of the depression at the start of the study, the magnitude of the effect of antidepressant treatment was constant: the effect on the placebo-controlled groups was lower the higher the initial depression score. The difference between the effects of the drug and the placebo was statistically significant only in the case of severe depression (a score greater than 28) (Kirsch et al. 2008).

In the words of Kirsch:

Drug-placebo differences in antidepressant efficacy increase as a function of baseline severity, but are relatively small even for severely depressed patients. The relationship between initial severity and antidepressant efficacy is attributable to decreased responsiveness to placebo among very severely depressed patients, rather than to increased responsiveness to medication.

Kirsch and his collaborators were not alone in their observations, and many other researchers agreed with them. The FDA data and the meta-analysis of 45 trials in Phases 2 and 3 suggested there was most often a significant difference between the effects of antidepressants and placebos when they were used on patients suffering from severe forms of depression. Patients with a high HRSD score were less affected by the placebo, and the difference between the treatment and the placebo effect was significantly greater (Khan et al. 2002). An independent study of antidepressant trials of the FDA-approved drugs confirmed that the difference between the treatment and control groups essentially depended on the initial score of the patients. The score difference became clinically significant when the initial score was greater than 25 (Fournier et al. 2010). Finally, given the extensive critical evaluation of SSRIs, surprisingly there has been no recent systematic review of TCAs by the Cochrane Collaboration. It did, however, carry out a meta-analysis of the large amount of data available on amitriptyline The results obtained showed that amitriptyline, when compared with a placebo or no treatment, is an effective antidepressant even in cases of severe depression, but not without various side effects (Leucht et al. 2012).

Kirsch's results were criticised in 2010 by Fountoulakis, who maintained that his conclusions were not supported by the methodology of his meta-analysis. Since then, however, Kirsch has verified his procedures and analysis with a thorough review and a complete recalculation (Huedo-Medina et al. 2012). But the controversy between Fountoulakis and Kirsch did not end there, and in (2013) Fountoulakis published a further meta-analysis to refute Kirsch's conclusions. In it he states that "antidepressants are clearly superior to the placebo" and criticises the British guidelines produced by NICE, which do not suggest antidepressants as the first choice for treating mild or moderate depression (Fountoulakis et al. 2013).

Even Vöhringer and his collaborators, who were critical of Kirsch's results, found in their reanalysis of the FDA trials that antidepressants are not effective for mild depression, that only acute treatment with them is effective for serious cases, and that the long-term effectiveness of this acute treatment remains unproven (Vöhringer and Ghaemi 2011). Ghaemi and his collaborators agreed that the effectiveness of antidepressants in the long term remains uncertain. They also suggested that their limited effectiveness is partially attributable to unrealistic expectations about their healing properties. According to these authors the expectations of antidepressants need to be reconsidered, and they suggested a revival of the concept of neurotic depression for mild or moderate cases. They also suggested possibly associating episodic or chronic mood disorders with anxiety, and therefore revising the DSM's diagnostic criteria (Ghaemi 2008).

Interestingly, numerous scientific reviews, including the *Annals of General Psychiatry*, require authors who publish articles to declare possible conflicts of interest. In his 2013 article in the *Annals of General Psychiatry*, Fountoulakis stated: "Competing interests: support concerning travel and accommodation expenses from various pharmaceutical companies in order to participate in medical congresses, honoraria for lectures from AstraZeneca, Janssen-Cilag, Eli Lilly *and a research grant from the Pfizer Foundation*."[8] Scientific reviews ask for this kind of declaration in order to uncover possible conflicts of interest which could influence the publication and even lead to bias.

Possible biases that could affect the validity of clinical trial results have become an increasingly serious problem, and it is worthwhile delving into some examples. In 2003, Melander analysed the studies submitted to the Swedish regulatory body to authorise treatments for major depressive disorder. These studies were also selectively published in scientific journals in order to influence the results. Melander concluded that "any attempt to recommend a specific selective serotonin reuptake inhibitor from the publicly available data only is likely to be based on biased evidence" (Melander et al. 2003). In the same year, Baker published a paper in which he observed that, in studies comparing TCAs with SSRIs, there were better results for the latter in the studies sponsored by their manufacturers (Baker et al. 2003). A similar study was recently conducted in the USA comparing current FDA data with published information. An examination of the drug efficacy papers published in scientific journals showed that 94% had positive results, compared to 51% in the FDA data. The authors concluded that because of the behaviour of antidepressant manufacturers, "selective reporting of clinical trials may have adverse consequences for researchers, study participants, health care professionals and patients" (Turner et al. 2008).

There have also been potential conflicts of interest in relation to the drafting of editions of the DSM, largely to do with the groups of specialists working on the various different categories of disorder. In the case of the DSM-IV-TR, 56% of the 170 panel members had financial ties to the pharmaceutical industry, and this figure rose to 100% for specialists working on mood disorders, schizophrenia and other psychotic disorders. The study concluded by recommending that the DSM request that anyone working on diagnostic categories that led to the prescription of drugs produced by profit-driven entities declare their financial ties (Cosgrove et al. 2006).

The controversy was rekindled in 2014, when the DSM requested that everyone involved in drafting the diagnostic categories of the DSM-5 declare any possible conflicts of interest. An interesting study examined the clinical trials of drugs for mental disorders defined by the new diagnostic categories. It found that 61% of the members of the DSM Task Force and 27% of the members of the Work Group reported financial conflicts of interest. Meanwhile, 38% of the principal investigators reported conflicts of interest, and 23% of these were also panel members who had decision-making authority on the DSM-5. The study concluded that the APA's mandatory disclosure of conflicts of interest for DSM-5 panel members may "not be robust enough to prevent the appearance of bias in both the DSM revision process as well as clinical decisions about appropriate interventions for DSM disorders" (Cosgrove et al. 2014).

At this point it seems appropriate to discuss the usefulness of clinical trials for determining the effectiveness of antidepressant treatments, and the significance of the size of the score reduction in the HRSD. Each of the HRSD's 17 items has a score of 0–3 (from absent to clearly present, in items 4–6, 12–14 and 17), or from 0 to 5 (from absent to very severe, in items 1–3, 7–11 and 15–16) depending on the assessor's evaluation of the patient. But there are no clear, scientifically determined thresholds to assess severity. The APA suggests a score of between 8 and 13 for mild depression, 14 and 18 for moderate, 19 and 22 for severe, and over 22 for very severe (Rush 2000). There are other obvious limitations besides the lack of justification for these threshold values. For example, a one-point reduction in each of the three items to do with sleep will lead to an overall three-point reduction, which is enough to market an antidepressant in the UK, and well above the median 1.70 of the SSRIs authorised by the FDA. It's even more alarming when you consider that, using these criteria, hypnotic drugs for non-depressed patients suffering from sleep disorders can be classed as effective antidepressants (Penn and Tracy 2012).

It is important to note that, in general terms, the data published on antidepressants shows a statistically significant effect,[9] but one of only marginal clinical relevance (NICE 2004). The FDA does not approve treatments that cause *any* reduction on the HRSD; it must be above their threshold. The meta-analysis available suggests that SSRI antidepressants cause a significant reduction of 1.7 points compared to placebo-controlled groups (Moncrieff and Kirsch 2005). In the UK, the NICE guidelines require a three-point difference between the group treated with the drug and the placebo-controlled group (although, as noted earlier, this is no longer stated explicitly) (NICE 2009; Abraham and Davis 2009). The same applies to Global Clinical Impression (GCI) Scale scores, which are also used widely. A three-point reduction using the HRSD corresponds to a four-point score using the GCI Scale (Leucht et al. 2013).

Despite the large number of studies, meta-analyses and critical reviews published, the effectiveness and safety of antidepressants remains controversial. This led to a study called the Sequenced Treatment Alternatives to Relieve Depression (STAR*D), sponsored by the National Institute of Mental Health (NIMH) of the US National Institutes of Health (NIH)[10] (NIMH 2006). Launched in 2000, it was a 6-year comprehensive evaluation of antidepressant medication, costing 35 million dollars. Its organisers described it as the largest practical trial to examine the treatment of major depressive disorder with pharmacotherapy and cognitive behavioural psychotherapy. Its aim was to determine whether some treatments would be effective for patients whose initial treatments were unsuccessful (Sinyor et al. 2010).

Patients enrolled had to have been diagnosed with major depressive disorder according to the DSM criteria and have at least a 14-point score on the HRSD. These patients then received standard treatment with citalopram a second-generation SSRI. If the citalopram treatment was ineffective, however, patients were put on randomised trials with other treatments. These included changing drugs (switching, increased doses (augmentation therapy and the conjunction of more than one drug (combination therapy; one group was also treated with psychotherapy. The primary outcome measure was remission at the end of the treatment, which was assessed on the HRSD. The study did not use placebo-controlled groups, however, so in this sense it did not meet the RCT standard (Warden et al. 2007).

4041 subjects were initially enrolled on the study, including both institutionalised patients and outpatients from general medicine, free of psychotic symptoms. The results obtained from these patients were analysed extensively and were the subject of numerous publications and reviews (Gaynes et al. 2009). Overall, the results did not quite meet the expectations implied in the title 'STAR*D. Revising conventional wisdom' (Rush et al. 2009).

Essentially, for the initial steps of the study there was between 13% and 37% remission. The switching, augmentation and combination therapy strategies that followed did not produce significant results. Overall, the cognitive behavioural psychotherapy was more effective than pharmacotherapy (Rush et al. 2009).

These unsettling results were so significant that they led the Director of NIMH, Thomas Insel, to publish a series of observations on his blog on the NIMH website (Insel 2009). Insel notes that, first and foremost, the study constitutes:

> … a new approach to clinical trials as part of an NIMH effort to support research with direct, practical value to clinicians. These trials, variously called "practical trials" or "effectiveness trials," differ from traditional efficacy trials in several ways. Whereas traditional efficacy trials have strict inclusion criteria, usually compare a drug against placebo, and limit outcome to rating scales, effectiveness trials include a broad spectrum of patients (including suicidal patients in depression trials), compare active

trials rather than active treatment against placebo, and focus on real-world outcomes such as measures of functioning. In addition, these new trials often test effectiveness with self-declared patients in primary care settings where most depressed patients receive treatment. Traditional efficacy trials generally study symptomatic volunteers recruited via advertisements, and the setting is either in academic health centers or commercial clinical research organisations.

Insel concludes:

> From Phase 1[11] it appears that the SSRI citalopram is only sufficient for a minority of patients, particularly high-functioning, well-educated women with few comorbid psychiatric or medical problems. Since there was no placebo control group, we do not know how many of these patients would remit without active drug treatment, so even for this 30%, can we be certain of the value of the drug? This trial was not designed to test efficacy of citalopram treatment, for which comparable remission rates with SSRIs in placebo-controlled, 8-week, randomised, controlled trials had already been reported. But the bigger question is how to choose the treatment for the other 70% of patients.

STAR*D has examined this and it is interesting to note the criticisms levelled against current protocols.

STAR*D made remarkable criticisms of current antidepressants, but this same study and the papers reporting it also encountered significant criticism themselves. In 2015 Peter Gøtzsche, a respected Danish researcher and cofounder of the Cochrane Collaboration, published a book on psychiatric drugs. One chapter of it is entitled 'STAR*D study: a case of consumer fraud?' In it, he points to what he considers numerous and serious scientific mistakes in the preparation of the study and in the papers reporting its results. In his opinion, this led to unjustified optimistic conclusions about the effectiveness of antidepressants (Goetzsche 2015).

NIMH's efforts to return to a realistic approach, strongly grounded in the reality of mental suffering and its treatment, are not limited to depression. Alongside STAR*D, NIMH also carried out a similar study for bipolar disorder (BD, which we have already come across under previous names such as cyclothymia and manic depression). It was called STEP-BD and the CATIE study of schizophrenia. The results obtained from STEP-BD, which concern depression in bipolar patients, correspond with those obtained from STAR*D and so will not be considered further. At the same time, the limitations of the current clinical trials for authorising new antidepressants and other medicines are obvious.

Thomas Insel recently returned to the subject of depression treatment, and reported on his blog that NIMH had made significant changes to the financing of clinical trials (Insel 2014). Insel affirms that:

> … we are taking the first step in an initiative that aims to realign research – but this time, the target is treatment development, an area in which progress has been frustratingly slow. In a series of funding announcements, NIMH is making three important changes to how we will fund clinical trials.

> First, future trials will follow an experimental medicine approach in which interventions serve not only as potential treatments, but as probes to generate information about the mechanisms underlying a disorder … a subset of the funding will support clinical trials that evaluate the effectiveness or increase the clinical impact of pharmacological, somatic, psychosocial, rehabilitative and combinative interventions.

> Second, future trials will need to meet new standards for efficiency, transparency and reporting … with new requirements for timelines, trial registration, publication and data sharing.

> Third, to ensure that these new requirements become the norm and not the exception, we will not support new clinical trials under past funding announcements … new trials will be reviewed according to these new criteria, which include target engagement and new performance metrics.

> Why these changes to our clinical trials enterprise? Treatment development has stalled. The pharmaceutical industry pipeline for medications is depleted, after several decades of "me-too" drugs. … Over the past decade, NIMH has supported large-scale, expensive effectiveness trials, such as CATIE and STAR*D. These trials were useful for identifying the limits of current treatments, but not helpful for improving outcomes … we will be shifting to trials that focus on trials as a way of defining the

next generation of treatments. The goal is better outcomes, measured as improved real-world functioning as well as reduced symptoms.

Insel and NIMH's vision of abandoning the empirical approach to developing new antidepressants and replacing it with an approach based on modern scientific principles is encouraging. According to these new guidelines, institutions should adopt realistic criteria for assessing the efficacy of drugs, and should also study drug targets. This will be done by including significant biomarkers while also making the most of modern neuroscience research techniques, including biochemical and genetic-molecular methods. Details of these techniques will be outlined in the following chapters.

Notes

1. A "blockbuster" is a medicine that generates annual sales of at least one billion dollars.
2. When Newsweek's Dokoupil presented Andrea Tone's book, The Age of Anxiety, the report estimated that one billion meprobamate pills had been sold, one-third of all pills sold at that time (Dokoupil 2010).
3. Emphasis added by the author.
4. Individual items are scored for each patient and the total is the measure of the severity of the depression.
5. The inclusion of a subject in a study or trial.
6. These drugs can be referred to by the exact chemical name of their active ingredient (complex, rarely used), or by the generic name given to them (a type of chemical name simplified for current use), or by the name of a generic drug (there may be several different names for the same active ingredient in different countries, or when different pharmaceutical forms are on the market for different methods of administration). Sometimes the simplified name of the chemical class they fall under (i.e. BDZ for anxiolytics, phenothiazine for antipsychotics) is used.
7. MAO-A is located mainly in the nervous system, and MAO-B is mainly present outside it.
8. Emphasis added by the author.

9. Verified repeatedly and not at random.
10. The NIH are an enormous federal structure in the USA, whose campus at Bethesda, Maryland comprises 27 institutes specialising in specific illnesses; among these is the NIMH. The NIH are the largest financers of extramural research, with grants totalling 31 billion dollars in 2010.
11. Of the STAR*D.

References

Abraham, J., & Davis, C. (2009). Drug evaluation and the permissive principle continuities and contradictions between standards and practices in antidepressant regulation. *Social Studies of Science, 39*(4), 569–598.

Adams, C. P., & Brantner, V. V. (2006). Estimating the cost of new drug development: Is it really $802 Million? *Health Affairs, 25*(2), 420–429.

Adams, C. P., & Brantner, V. V. (2010). Spending on new drug development. *Health Economy, 19*(2), 130–141.

Baker, C. B., Johnsrud, M. T., Crismon, M. L., et al. (2003). Quantitative analysis of sponsorship bias in economic studies of antidepressants. *British Journal of Psychiatry, 183,* 498–506.

Beck, J. S. (1995). *Cognitive therapy: Basics and beyond.* New York: The Guilford Press.

Bracken, M. B. (2013). *Risk, chance and causation. Investigating the origins and treatment of diseases.* New Haven: Yale University Press.

Brunton, L., Lazo, J., & Parker, K. (2005). *Goodman & Gilman's, The pharmacological basis of therapeutics* (11th ed.). New York: McGraw-Hill Medical.

Cochrane. (2016). *Cochrane. Trusted evidence. Informed decisions. Better health.* n.d. http://www.cochrane.org/about-us Accessed 30 May 2016.

Cosgrove, L., Krimsky, S., Vijayaraghavan, M., et al. (2006). Financial ties between DSM-IV panel members and the pharmaceutical industry. *Psychotherapy and Psychosomatics, 75*(3), 154–160.

Cosgrove, L., Krimsky, S., Wheeler, E. E., et al. (2014). Tripartite conflicts of interest and high Stakes Patent Extensions in the DSM-5. *Psychotherapy and Psychosomatics, 83*(2), 106–113.

Dokoupil, T. (2010). *America's long love affair with anti-anxiety drugs.* http://www.newsweek.com/americas-long-love-affair-anti-anxiety-drugs-77967. Accessed 25 March 2015.

Elmore, J. G., & Feinstein, A. R. (1994). Joseph Goldberger: An unsung hero of American clinical epidemiology. *Annals of Internal Medicine, 121*(5), 372–375.

FDA. (1997). *Guidance for industry. Guidance for the clinical evaluation of antidepressant drugs.* Center for Drug Evaluation and Research. U.S. Department of Health and Human Services, Food and Drug Administration. U.S. Food and Drug Administration. Protecting and promoting your health. http://www.fda.gov/downloads/Drugs/GuidanceComplianceRegulatoryInformation/Guidances/ucm071299.pdf. Accessed 20 March 2014.

FDA. (2015). *List of antidepressants drugs with medication guides* http://www.fda.gov/downloads/Drugs/DrugSafety/InformationbyDrugClass/UCM161647.pdf. Accessed 2 February 2015.

Fountoulakis, K. N., Veroniki, A. A., Siamouli, M. et al. (2013). No role for initial severity on the efficacy of antidepressants: Results of a multi-meta-analysis. *Annals of General Psychiatry, 12*(1): 26–36. doi: 10.1186/1744-859X-12-26.

Fournier, J. C., DeRubeis, R. J., Hollon, S. D., et al. (2010). Antidepressant drug effects and depression severity. A patient-level meta-analysis. *The Journal of American Medical Association, 303*(1), 47–53.

Fung, M., Thornton, A., Mybeck, K., et al. (2001). Evaluation of the characteristics of safety withdrawal of prescription drugs from worldwide pharmaceutical markets 1960 to 1999. *Therapeutic Innovation & Regulatory Science, 35*(1), 293–317.

Gaynes, B. N., Warden, D., Trivedi, M. H., et al. (2009). What did STAR*D teach us? Results from a large-scale, practical, clinical trial for patients with depression. *Psychiatric Services, 60*(11), 1439–1445.

Ghaemi, S. N. (2008). Why antidepressants are not antidepressants: STEP-BD, STAR*D, and the return of neurotic depression. *Bipolar Disorders, 10*(8), 957–968.

Goetzsche, P. (2015). *Deadly psychiatry and organized denial.* København: People's Press.

Goozner, M. (2004). *The $800 million pill. The truth behind the cost of new drugs.* Oakland: University of California Press.

Hamilton, M. (1960). A rating scale for depression. *Journal of Neurology, Neurosurgery and Psychiatry, 23*, 56–62.

Hamilton, M. (1967). Development of a rating scale for primary depressive illness. *British Journal of Social and Clinical Psychology, 6*(4), 278–296.

Healy, D. (1997). *The antidepressant era.* Cambridge: Harvard University Press.

Huedo-Medina, T. B., Johnson, B. T., & Kirsch, I. (2012). Kirsch et al.'s (2008) calculations are correct: Reconsidering Fountoulakis & Moller's re-analysis of the Kirsch data. *International Journal of Neuropsychopharmacology, 15*(8), 1193–1198.

Insel, T. (2009). Beyond efficacy: The STAR*D Trial. National Institute of Mental Health (NIMH). http://www.nimh.nih.gov/about/director/bio/publications/beyond-efficacy-the-star-d-trial.shtml. Accessed 24 March 2014.

Insel, T. (2014). *Director's Blog: A new approach to clinical trials. National Institute of Mental Health.* Retrieved February 1, 2015, from http://www.nimh.nih.gov/about/director/2014/a-new-approach-to-clinical-trials.shtml.

Khan, A., Leventhal, R. M., Khan, S. R., et al. (2002). Severity of depression and response to antidepressants and placebo: An analysis of the food and drug administration database. *Journal of Clinical Psychopharmacology, 22*(1), 40–45.

Kirsch, I., Deacon, B. J., Huedo-Medina, T. B., Scoboria, A., Moore, T. J., & Johnson, B. T (2008). Initial severity and antidepressant benefits: A meta-analysis of data submitted to the Food and Drug Administration. *PLoS Medicine, 5*(2), e45. doi: 10.1371/journal.pmed.0050045 .

Kirsch, I., & Sapirstein, G. (1998). Listening to prozac but hearing placebo: A meta-analysis of antidepressant medication. Prevention & Treatment, *1*(0002a). http://dx.doi.org/10.1037/1522-3736.1.1.12a.

Leucht, C., Huhn, M., & Leucht, S. (2012). Amitriptyline versus placebo for major depressive disorder. *Cochrane Database of Systematic Reviews*, (12). doi: 10.1002/14651858.

Leucht, S., Fennema, H., Engel, R., et al. (2013). What does the HAMD means? *Journal of Affective Disorders, 148*(2–3), 243–248.

Melander, H., Ahlqvist-Rastad, J., Meijer, G., et al. (2003). Evidence b(i)ased medicine—selective reporting from studies sponsored by pharmaceutical industry: Review of studies in new drug applications. *British Medical Journal, 326*(7400), 1171–1173.

Moncrieff, J., & Kirsch, I. (2005). Efficacy of antidepressants in adults. *Britsh Medical Journal, 331*(7509), 155–159.

Mullin, R. (2014). Tufts study finds big rise in cost of drug development. *Chemical & Engineering News, 92*(47), p. 6. Retrieved February 1, 2015, from http://cen.acs.org/articles/92/i47/Tufts-Study-Finds-Big-Rise.html?type=paidArticleContent.

Murrough, J. W., & Charney, D. S. (2012). Is there anything really novel on the antidepressant horizon? *Current Psychiatry Reports, 14*(6), 643–649.

National Institute for Health and Care Excellence (NICE). (2004). Depression: Management of depression in primary and secondary care NICE guidelines [CG23]. Retrieved May 30, 2016, from https://www.nice.org.uk/guidance/cg23.

National Institute for Health and Care Excellence (NICE). (2009). Depression in adults: The treatment and management of depression in adults. Retrieved April 12, 2015, from https://www.nice.org.uk/guidance/cg90.

NIMH. (2006). Sequenced treatment alternatives to relieve depression (STAR*D). ClinicalTrials.gov, http://www.clinicaltrials.gov/ct/show/NCT-00021528?order=1. Accessed March 20, 2014.

Penn, E., & Tracy, D. K. (2012). The drug don't work? Antidepressants and the current and future pharmacological management of depression. *Therapeutic Advances in Psychopharmacology, 2*(5), 179–188.

Rush, A. J., First, M. B., & Blacker, D. (2000). *Handbook of psychiatric measures*. Washington, DC: American Psychiatric Press.

Rush, A. J., Warden, D., Wisniewski, S. R., et al. (2009). STAR*D. Revising Conventional Wisdom. *CNS Drugs, 23*(8), 627–647.

Shulman, K. I., Herrmann, N., & Walker, S. E. (2013). Current place of monoamine oxidase inhibitors in the treatment of depression. *CNS Drugs, 27*(10), 789–797.

Sinyor, M., Schaffee, A., & Levitt, A. (2010). The sequenced treatment alternatives to relieve depression (STAR*D) trial: A review. *La Revue Canadienne de Psychiatrie, 55*(3), 126–137.

Tone, A. (2009). *The age of anxiety: A history of America's turbulent affair with tranquilizers*. New York: Basic Books.

Turner, E. H., Matthews, A. M., Linardatos, E., et al. (2008). Selective publication of antidepressant trials and its influence on apparent efficacy. *New England Journal of Medicine, 358,* 252–260.

Vöhringer, P. A., & Ghaemi, S. N. (2011). Solving the antidepressant efficacy question: Effect sizes in major depressive disorder. *Clinical Therapeutics, 33*(12), B49–B61.

Warden, D., Rush, A. J., Trivedi, M. H., et al. (2007). The STAR*D project results: A comprehensive review of findings. *Current Psychiatry Reports, 9*(6), 449–459.

Wong, D. T., Perry, K. W., & Bymaster, F. P. (2005). The discovery of fluoxetine hydrochloride (Prozac). *Nature Reviews Drug Discovery, 4,* 764–774.

9

A Matter of Chemistry

A specialist is a man who knows more and more about less and less.
William J. Mayo

Rapid medical progress after the Second World War led to the identification of the mechanisms behind healthy and unhealthy brain function. The drugs and psychotropic substances that influence brain processes were also identified, and the foundations of modern psychopharmacology and antidepressants established. It was possible to show that psychotropic substances acted on the nervous system by interfering with neurotransmission, the basic mechanism of the nervous system, whereby neurones communicate with other neurones, or with the organs, muscles and glands controlled by them.

The first modern developments in this field were achieved by demonstrating that nerves and muscles are excitable tissues, and that excitation is a temporary change in the electric state, responsible for the nervous impulse and muscle contraction. It was also shown that in the vagus nerve, part of the parasympathetic nervous system—one of two divisions of the autonomic nervous system—the nerve impulse is transmitted along the nerve fibre to an involuntary muscle, which it

© The Author(s) 2017
T. Giraldi, *Unhappiness, Sadness and 'Depression'*,
DOI 10.1007/978-3-319-57657-2_9

controls by releasing a chemical messenger (acetylcholine). The process was named "neurotransmission", and acetylcholine was the neurotransmitter. Acetylcholine acts on the muscle by binding to specific structures (receptors) exposed at the nerve ending, causing muscle excitation. Then, at the end of the transmission process, acetylcholine is inactivated by enzyme breakdown.[1]

The chemist Otto Loewi discovered neurotransmission and the role of acetylcholine in 1921, and was awarded the 1936 Nobel Prize in Physiology and Medicine, along with Henry Hallett Dale (Nobel Prize in Physiology and Medicine 1936). Neurotransmitters were studied in greater depth in the following years, and this led to the identification of norepinephrine the neurotransmitter in the sympathetic nervous system, the other division of the autonomic nervous system. Its discovery is credited to the chemist Ulf von Euler, who was awarded the 1970 Nobel Prize in Physiology and Medicine, along with Julius Axelrod and Bernard Katz (Nobel Prize in Physiology and Medicine 1970).

Soon after the discovery of acetylcholine and norepinephrine neurotransmission, it was also found that neurones communicated through a contact point between the nerve fibre and the neurone cell body, in a specialised structure called the "synapsis". Studies using biochemical techniques also deepened our understanding of the subject and identified a number of new neurotransmitters[2] (López-Muñoz and Alamo 2009a).

The years following the middle of the last century saw a revolution in psychiatry. Scientists discovered the clinical applications of a number of vital molecules, including anxiolytics, antipsychotics, antidepressants and antimanic drugs. These compounds were so effective at alleviating the symptoms of mental illness that even after more than half a century they are still in use today, and serve as a standard of comparison to determine the efficacy and safety of new derivatives.

As the number of psychotropic drugs has grown, so too has our understanding of brain function, neurotransmitters and neurotransmission mechanisms, paving the way for a large amount of experimental research. This suggested that mental disorders were associated with alterations in neurotransmission (Mendels and Fraser 1974), and that symptoms were alleviated when these alterations were corrected

(López-Muñoz and Alamo 2009b; Belmaker and Agam 2008). This led to the rise of the chemical imbalance theory, which spread across the scientific community and even into the media. The theory was also reinforced when first-generation antidepressants were joined by selective serotonin reuptake inhibitors (SSRIs), whose extraordinary popularity turned them into a cultural phenomenon (Leo and Lacasse 2008).

According to the theory, moods depended on the brain's chemistry (McGeer and McGeer 1980; Castrén 2005), but it did not stop with moods: Young also envisaged reducing love to the results of neuroscientific investigation (Young 2009). A group of Italian researchers examined romantic love in particular, concluding that it was an obsessive compulsive disorder (among the mental disorders listed by the DSM) associated with abnormalities in the serotonin transporter, which is the target of SSRI action (Marazziti et al. 1999). In fact, this work received the 2000 Ig Nobel Prize (Ig Nobel Prize 2000), an award given annually by the scientific journal *Annals of Improbable Research* to researchers who carry out "strange, amusing, and lastly absurd research which makes people laugh and then think". It is awarded by the winners of the actual Nobel Prize in a public award ceremony at Harvard University.

Soon after Carlsson discovered dopamine in 1957, scientists related it to schizophrenia and its response to new antipsychotic drugs (Bennett 1998). A large number of experimental studies were also carried out into the role of norepinephrine and serotonin in mood disorders, which led to the monoamine theory of depression.[3] We still have a large amount of information about the history of this theory (Mulinari 2012; Wrobel 2007), so it is possible to look at the evidence behind it in detail.

It is tempting to believe the theory that depressive disorder is caused by a neurotransmitter deficiency, and that antidepressants (such as tricyclics and monoamine oxidase inhibitors) are effective because they correct this. The idea was first proposed in a historic and much-cited (1965) article by Schildkraut on the effects of reserpine and antidepressants. Schildkraut firmly believed that catecholamines, and particularly norepinephrine, played a significant part in affective disorders, and stated that "monoamine oxidase inhibitors increase brain concentrations of norepinephrine while imipraminelike agents potentiate the physiological effects of norepinephrine. Reserpine, a drug which can cause clinical depression, depletes catecholamines." He does, however, recognise that "[c]linical studies relevant to the catecholamine hypothesis are limited and the findings are inconclusive" (Schildkraut 1965).

As Schildkraut observed, the initial evidence was essentially based on the properties of reserpine. As mentioned earlier, reserpine is a natural substance contained in the medicinal plant *Rauwolfia serpentina* and used in traditional Indian medicine to treat snake bites, fever and mental disorders. It was first used in Western medicine in the early 1950s as an antihypertensive and antipsychotic (Magarian 1991). Reserpine acts by interfering with norepinephrine and dopamine, which are stored in the vesicles, released by nerve impulses into the synaptic cleft and taken back up into the nerve fibre and vesicles through impulse transmission. The reuptake process would prove crucial for the effective functioning of the monoaminergic synapses, which are responsible for the concentration of neurotransmitters in the synaptic cleft and for returning the synapses to their original state after the transmission of the nerve impulse.[4]

Reserpine works by blocking the vesicles' monoamine transporter, keeping monoamines out and allowing them to be degraded by the monoamine oxidases. Reserpine thus markedly reduces their concentration in the nerve endings. This is the basis for reserpine's antihypertensive action, in as far as it inhibits the sympathetic component of the autonomic nervous system. In psychiatric patients, this has both sedative and antipsychotic effects. Because of the growing theory that schizophrenia is caused by neurotransmission disturbances, these effects are often attributed to the depletion of the neurotransmitter dopamine.

The use of reserpine in psychiatry was short-lived, however, and it was quickly replaced by chlorpromazine and haloperidol, which could selectively reduce psychotic symptoms without a sedative effect. One of reserpine's properties seemed clear, however: its ability to cause adverse effects and depress the nervous system in hypertensive patients. It was found that the same was true of other drugs that inhibited the sympathetic component and reached the brain, like methyldopa clonidine and beta-blockers their antihypertensive action was also accompanied by a sedative effect (Beers and Passman 1990).

This is understandable when you consider that there is a high concentration of the neurotransmitter norepinephrine in the principal brain system, the locus ceruleus, which regulates attention, brain activation (arousal) and stress responses (Benarroch 2009). As a result, it's possible to see how reserpine and other antihypertensive inhibitors that reduce the available quantity of norepinephrine cause a marked sedative effect. In the case of reserpine, it not only worked as a sedative but also induced real depression that became widespread and firmly rooted. Animals were even experimented on with reserpine to study depression and antidepressants. A more thorough examination of the drug, however, showed that in general it does not induce depression, although it can have this effect on people who have previously suffered from depression or are particularly vulnerable to it. It was its effects on these groups that gave rise to the myth that reserpine is a depressogenic. This has contributed to the widespread reluctance to abandon the alluring monoamine-based hypothesis that "is still of great importance. It serves as a heuristic to guide research, it enhances psychiatry's prestige, and it helps to validate and promote drug therapy for depression." (Baumeister et al. 2003).

Extensive research was then carried out into the question of whether a deficit of brain monoamines was at the root of depression, and if antidepressants could correct this deficit.[5] But scientists immediately encountered the methodological problem of how to measure the concentration of norepinephrine in the nervous system. The neurotransmitter's physiological role is in the synaptic cleft, so it's here that a shortage would be found: the internal structure where the nerve ending transmits impulses to the body of neurones. Not only is this structure miniscule, inside it neurotransmission occurs within just a few thousandths of a second. In addition, only a tiny fraction of the billions of neurones that make up the brain are involved in mood disorders. Because there were no techniques for gaining direct access to the synaptic cleft, all studies published at the time had to use indirect measurements, such as the amount of neurotransmitters diffusing into the area outside the synaptic cleft, or the neurotransmitter levels in biological fluids such as urine, plasma and the cerebrospinal fluid of the central nervous system.

Yet another complication was that, before neurotransmitters could reach these various biochemical fluids, they had to undergo enzyme degradation, so all that could be measured were metabolic products. The concentration of homovanillic acid (HVA) was therefore measured, because this is a product of the degradation of dopamine and norepinephrine. 5-hydroxyindoleacetic acid (5-HIAA) was also measured as a by-product of the degradation of serotonin.

The relationship between dopamine and both schizophrenia and antipsychotics was therefore being clearly established. Dopamine only plays a marginal role in depression, however, so it will not be examined further in this book. Studies of norepinephrine and serotonin, on the other hand, would play a key role in understanding mood disorders.

Despite researchers' best efforts, studies into the levels of HVA and 5-HIAA did not conclusively show significant deficiencies of dopamine, norepinephrine and serotonin in mentally ill patients (Bowers et al. 1969; Papeschi and McClure 1971), or in psychiatric patients prior to pharmacotherapeutic treatment (Bowers 1974; Maas et al. 1984).

Studies into the monoaminergic hypothesis of depression and antidepressants did gain significant and relevant results, however, through in vitro and animal experimentation. It was found that the reuptake of norepinephrine could be inhibited by imipramine and tricyclic antidepressants (Glowinski and Axelrod 1964; Lahti and Maickel 1971; Ross and Renyi 1967). Antidepressants were also found to inhibit serotonin reuptake (Ross and Renyi 1969).

It's important to underscore the fact that the initial evidence for a norepinephrine serotonin and dopamine reuptake mechanism, and for the inhibition of this mechanism by tricyclics, was obtained through in vitro models and animal experimentation. It was therefore crucial to determine whether this held true in a clinical setting, and the only way to do this was by measuring the concentration of metabolic degradation products in biological fluids. The researchers made great efforts, but they failed to find a significant correlation between the clinical response to tricyclic antidepressants and the levels of HVA and 5-HIAA in patients' biological fluids (Bowers 1974).

Other researchers even considered the urinary elimination of a product that "could reflect the metabolism of norepinephrine in the human brain",[6] but reported complex results that still showed no direct relationship between an antidepressant response and the urinary metabolite levels, and did not uphold the "hypothesis about the association of alterations in serotonin and norepinephrine and *definable subtypes*[7] of depression" (Maas et al. 1984).

The hypothesis that depression is caused by a lack of norepinephrine and serotonin in the brain, and that tricyclic antidepressants act to correct this deficiency, came to be accepted as a theory based on sound scientific evidence. The properties of monoamine oxidase inhibitors seemed to support this theory: the inhibition of the enzyme caused the neurotransmitter to undergo a limited enzymatic degradation in the nerve fibre, causing it to be present in greater quantities, limiting the initial deficit (Racagni and Popoli 2008). But, in fact, the evidence for this was fleeting and indirect and did not support the initial hypothesis.

The theory that the lack of norepinephrine and serotonin in people suffering from depression could be corrected with tricyclic antidepressants was initially based on the notion that reserpine had a depressogenic effect on those not suffering from mental disorders. But the problem with this was differentiating between a sedative state and actual depressive suffering; these conditions actually share a number of traits. This problem, which actually also affects the assessment of a number of drugs, still remains today.

The first point that contradicts the monoaminergic theory of depression arises from the effects of reserpine on both depressed and anxious patients. A study was conducted into the matter in Davies and Shepherd (1955) and, despite the fact that it preceded the diffusion of evidence-based medicine and randomised controlled clinical trials its methodology was incontrovertible even by today's standards. The results clearly showed that reserpine had significant anxiolytic and antidepressant effects, accompanied by both modest and toxic side effects (Davies and Shepherd 1955). Substances that cause an even more marked reduction of catecholamines than reserpine, however, such as 6-hydroxydopamine, alpha-methyl-para-tyrosine and para-chlorophenylalanine (which have not been used clinically), do not also induce depressive states (Mendels and Frazer 1974).

Another characteristic of antidepressants that has been reported since they first began to be used is the latency of their effects. The full antidepressant action occurs after 1 or 2 weeks of treatment; the synaptic transporters of monoamine are inhibited almost instantaneously: numerous theories have been proposed to account for the time difference (Racagni and Popoli 2008; Svensson 2000).

Other psychotropic substances were examined in conjunction with tricyclic antidepressants, with interesting results. Cocaine was shown to inhibit the reuptake of monoamine in a similar way to tricyclic antidepressants; amphetamine was found to replace the nerve impulse by inducing the release of the neurotransmitter from the nerve ending (Rothman et al. 2001; Sulzer et al. 2005). Cocaine and amphetamine have action mechanisms that cause similar synaptic effects to antidepressants, but they are not as effective. Unlike antidepressants, they intensely stimulate the nervous system and quickly cause severe addiction. Failed attempts to apply them to psychiatry led to their abandonment in therapy (Karch 1999; Rasmussen 2008), and instead they were widely abused and often used in doping; now they fall under antidrug legislation. On a related note, the study of the structure-activity relationship of cocaine has led to the development of local anaesthetics (Ruetsch et al. 2001), and of methylphenidate (Ritalin) from amphetamine. The drug is still used in the paediatric treatment of attention deficit hyperactive disorder (ADHD), causing considerable controversy (Baughman 2006).

After initial attempts, the study of the action mechanisms of antidepressants was soon bolstered by new biochemical techniques based on the use of tissues, their subcellular preparations, isolated organs and animal experimentation. The techniques involved marking the presence of adrenaline or serotonin with radioactive isotopes. Using these studies, it became possible to show that tricyclic antidepressants inhibit the reuptake of norepinephrine and serotonin. But conclusive proof that this was responsible for correcting a deficit, and that this deficit caused depressive disorders, remained elusive. It also remained uncertain whether norepinephrine or serotonin was involved in the supposed antidepressant action.

Studies into the action mechanisms of tricyclic antidepressants showed that all these compounds inhibited the reuptake of norepinephrine and serotonin, and the degree of inhibition depended on the antidepressant being studied. The selectivity drugs could be expressed with a number that indicated the ratio between the drug concentrations necessary to inhibit each transporter to the same extent. But the idea that the selectivity factor of each tricyclic antidepressant could be identified easily seemed immediately problematic.

During their clinical use, imipramine and amitriptyline underwent in vivo biotransformation, which inactivated them and facilitated their renal elimination. The intermediates produced in the process were pharmacologically active compounds: desipramine and nortriptyline. These compounds were found to be so active that they were quickly marketed as antidepressants; in fact, it was discovered that when imipramine and amitriptyline were used, these compounds contributed significantly to the magnitude of the response observed. Imipramine and amitriptyline inhibit the reuptake of norepinephrine and serotonin in practically the same way; nortriptyline, however, inhibits norepinephrine ten times more than serotonin, and desipramine almost 100 times more (Humble 2000). This data appears to indicate that antidepressant compounds mainly act to inhibit the reuptake of norepinephrine.

The synthesis of new molecules and the progress of neuroscience have helped with the problem of antidepressant inhibition selectivity. Psychopharmacological techniques were enriched by the use of synaptosomes. These are essentially subcellular preparations of neurones from the nervous systems of animals, which were used with in vitro biochemical techniques to study the functioning of synapses. Other studies included the examination of the platelet, a neurone model from the peripheral blood.

As psychopharmacology rapidly developed in this period, we also gained a deeper understanding of serotonin and its role as a modulator in a wide range of neurocognitive processes. It was linked to processes including mood, perception, memory, rage, aggression and fear, as well as stress, appetite, addiction and abuse, and sexual responses. It was also shown to be involved in motor control, regulation of the cerebellum, circadian rhythms, sleep, the tone of cerebral vessels, vomiting, breathing and temperature regulation, not forgetting the regulation of a myriad of vegetative functions outside the central nervous system (Berger et al. 2009).

It is therefore understandable that there was immediate interest in resolving serotonin's role in depression. One of the methods used was the manipulation of the amino acid tryptophan. It is an essential tool because it is not synthesised in organisms but has to be acquired through diet, and it is needed for the synthesis of serotonin in brain neurones. But when patients were given a limited tryptophan diet, although this caused a depletion of serotonin, it was not observed to cause significant mood deterioration (Delgado et al. 1994).

Another approach was to administer tryptophan to depressed subjects in order to increase serotonin levels and improve their moods. But the difference was so limited and doubtful that treatment with tryptophan, even when combined with antidepressants, now falls under the umbrella of so-called complementary and alternative medicine (CAM) (Mendels 1974; Ravindran and da Silva 2013). Overall, these studies did not help to determine the role of serotonin in depression.

In contrast, the development of new antidepressants did have a significant impact. Unlike tricyclics, new antidepressants like fluoxetine selectively inhibited serotonin reuptake. Fluoxetine was first mentioned in a 1974 publication, and Eli Lilly obtained FDA authorisation for its marketing in 1987 under the name Prozac. In 1975 the antidepressant market was estimated at a little over 200 million dollars, but with the arrival of fluoxetine, sales quickly began to soar, exceeding two billion dollars by 1995. By 1999, the American magazine *Fortune* was calling fluoxetine one of the "Pharmaceutical Products of the Century". By the time its patent expired, it had been prescribed to over 40 million patients and made a total of over 22 billion dollars in sales, with an annual peak of 2.8 billion in 1998 (Wong et al. 2005).

As more and more people started using fluoxetine, more and more studies were undertaken to investigate its properties. As far as its action mechanism is concerned, precise experimental studies confirmed that it selectively inhibited serotonin reuptake. However, these studies did not provide direct evidence that treatment with fluoxetine or tricyclic antidepressants corrected a serotonin-based neurotransmission deficit in the brain synapses. Efficacy studies also showed that, although it did not affect norepinephrine neurotransmission, fluoxetine was an effective antidepressant according to the current diagnostic criteria for depression, with all the criticisms associated with them.

Before discussing these issues, it is important to look briefly at the other SSRIs that were brought onto the market after fluoxetine. The success of fluoxetine showed that there was a lucrative market for antidepressants, and other pharmaceutical companies quickly became interested in SSRIs and the development of new compounds. In addition to fluoxetine, sertraline, paroxetine, fluvoxamine, citalopram and escitalopram were all approved for market. The selectivity of serotonin reuptake by sertraline, paroxetine and fluvoxamine was around 100 times greater than norepinephrine, and in the case of citalopram and escitalopram the ratio was 1000:1.

The discovery of a new molecule often leads to the study of its structure-activity relationship. The compound's structure is generally optimised to create new safer and more effective derivatives. The new SSRIs did not differ substantially from fluoxetine in terms of their efficacy, and all SSRIs cause much less pronounced adverse effects than tricyclic antidepressants. The new SSRIs, which are roughly equivalent to fluoxetine in terms of clinical response and adverse effects, were essentially authorised for market because the regulatory bodies only demanded that they were more effective than a placebo. The aim of the pharmaceutical companies who invested in producing new SSRIs does not seem to have been to gain a market share by producing innovative new active ingredients but rather by occupying parts of the existing market with medicines essentially similar to those already available, giving rise to the nickname "me-too" drugs.

This situation is described in great detail by Marcia Angell in her book *The Truth About the Drug Companies: How They Deceive Us and What to Do About It.* Angell's authoritativeness derives from her position as editor-in-chief of the prestigious *New England Journal of Medicine* from 1988 to 2000. As the first woman to have this honour, in 1997, *Time* magazine numbered her among the 25 most influential Americans (Angell 2004).

Citalopram, which was a particular success on the market, deserves special consideration. The citalopram molecule is composed of two identical molecular forms, and citalopram is a mix of the two. But when the patent expired and citalopram was expected to become much less profitable, it was much less expensive for the pharmaceutical company to analyse the properties of the two different forms and just use the form with the better properties. As a result, when the patent expired and citalopram became an "equivalent"[8] and less profitable product, one of the forms—escitalopram—was put on the market alone. Fortunately, it proved to have very similar properties to the original compound. This method allowed pharmaceutical companies to keep their medicines profitable after their patents expired, even if the drugs they marketed boasted very little in the way of innovation. It's a method that is now in widespread use for other drugs (Angell 2004).

The number of studies published on SSRIs after the introduction of fluoxetine to the market has been startling. A search in the PubMed database of the National Library of Medicine, US National Institutes of Health, indicates that over 40,000 studies on SSRIs were published from 1969 to 2013, of which almost 8000 were to do with clinical trials. The number of studies each year has grown progressively: from 1969–1974 there were about 100 per year, reaching 500 per year by 1990 and peaking at about 2000 per year between 2003 and 2013. In the same period, the number of studies per year to do with trials was about 30 in the early 1970s, rising to 100 in the 1990s and exceeding 400 between 2003 and 2013. The results from numerous clinical trials made it possible to extend SSRIs to other disorders beyond depression, including anxiety disorders, obsessive compulsive disorders and food disorders. Their less pronounced side effects have also led them to be used to treat other "off-label"[9] disorders.

Along with SSRIs, other new antidepressants, with different selectivity characteristics, were also developed to inhibit the synaptic reuptake of neurotransmitters. They were identified with a range of new acronyms. To name but a few: reboxetine, a selective norepinephrine reuptake inhibitor (NRI), as well as the serotoninnorepinephrine reuptake inhibitors (SNRIs) venlafaxine and duloxetine. Newer antidepressants have complex action mechanisms that include interactions with other cellular and molecular targets, such as the receptors for a range of neurotransmitters (Noradrenergic and specific serotonergic antidepressants, Serotonin antagonist and reuptake inhibitors and atypical ones); bupropion also has a complex action that includes the inhibition of dopamine reuptake (Racagni and Popoli 2008). Tianeptine is a particularly curious compound; chemically speaking it is a tricyclic derivative, produced by the French pharmaceutical company Servier and marketed outside France, but not in the USA and the UK. In the 1980s and 1990s there was a great deal of interest in tianeptine's action mechanism, which initial studies showed involved the stimulation of serotonin reuptake, which was in stark contrast to SSRIs. As a result, it was given the acronym SSRE (selective serotonin reuptake enhancer) (Brink et al. 2006). Later studies have indicated that its action mechanism involves complex neurobiological neurotransmitter mechanisms. The compound is an atypical antidepressant, and it is particularly interesting because of its pharmacological properties (McEwen et al. 2010).

The majority of clinical studies published lend themselves to a meta-analytical examination. One such examination aimed to determine the efficacy and acceptability of 12 of the new generation of antidepressants. It was carried out by a group of expert researchers and published in the reputable medical journal *The Lancet* in Cipriani et al. (2009). The authors selected 117 randomised controlled trials with a total of over 25,000 patients affected by major depression. These patients were treated with SSRIs (fluoxetine sertraline, fluvoxamine, paroxetine, citalopram and escitalopram), an NRI (reboxetine), SNRIs (duloxetine and venlafaxine) and two atypical compounds. The conclusions drawn were that "important differences exist between commonly prescribed antidepressants for both efficacy and acceptability in favour of escitalopram and sertraline. Sertraline might be the best choice when starting treatment for moderate to severe major depression in adults because it has the most favourable balance between benefits, acceptability and acquisition cost" (Cipriani et al. 2009).

Another authoritative study on antidepressants is the meta-analysis comparing the drugs used in psychiatry (16 drugs for eight psychiatric disorders) with those used in general medicine (48 drugs for 20 illnesses). The study found that, although some drugs in general medicine cause more pronounced effects than psychotropic agents, psychiatric drugs are generally no less effective than other drugs. Antidepressants caused a score reduction of more than three points on the Hamilton Rating Scale for Depression and a higher percentage of patients responded to them without side effects[10] (Leucht et al. 2012).

It's also important to consider reboxetine in light of an important article published in 2010 by the authoritative *British Medical Journal*. It was prefaced by a serious editorial and followed by a number of letters sent to the journal by alarmed readers. The meta-analysis focused on studies into the treatment of major depression in adults, and used only double-blind, randomised controlled trials lasting for at least 6 weeks. They had to have been published in scientific journals, available from publicly accessible sources, or be unpublished but available through the producer (Pfizer). The drug used was reboxetine (an NRI). The data of 3003 of the 4098 patients assessed was not published: reboxetine did not cause significant differences compared to the placebo, and the magnitude of the effects of reboxetine was inferior to the SSRIs fluoxetine paroxetine and citalopram The adverse effects were also more pronounced than those caused by SSRIs. The study concluded that "reboxetine is, overall, an ineffective and potentially harmful antidepressant. Published evidence is affected by publication bias, underlining the urgent need for mandatory publication of trial data" (Eyding et al. 2010).

When the data from all the clinical trials—which had been kept confidential by the sponsoring companies—was examined, a very different picture emerged to what was published in scientific journals. It is impossible to generalise, but there are ways in which the case of reboxetine recalls Kirsch's work, which included the confidential data from the clinical trials on SSRIs. Both cases also led to a growing demand for the results from all clinical trials on medicinal products to be made public.[11]

The effectiveness of the antidepressants on the market therefore seems limited and uncertain, and the next chapter will examine their safety in detail. Despite the accuracy of *in vitro* studies on the action mechanisms of antidepressants, the clinical data obtained does not help to decisively determine whether depression is caused by an actual chemical imbalance in the synapses, and whether that in turn is related to serotonin.

Leo and Lacasse have investigated the role of the media in the chemical imbalance theory of depression. Their starting point was that, although the causes of mental disorders such as depression are unknown, the pharmaceutical industry and members of the psychiatric profession vigorously promote the idea that depression is caused by a neurotransmitter imbalance. They then examined the media that reported the chemical imbalance theory, and asked authors and producers on what evidence they based their convictions. They also asked psychiatrists, patients and an important pharmaceutical company what evidence they had for the chemical imbalance theory. The evidence provided was neither adequate nor convincing, and many professionals stated firmly that the serotonin imbalance theory was known to be wrong. The authors concluded that the media could have a positive impact on mental health by ensuring they provide information congruent with relevant scientific journals (Leo and Lacasse 2008).

In 2005, these same authors published a work on the separation of advertising data from the available scientific literature. It should be remembered that direct-to-consumer advertising is only authorised in the USA; in other countries medicines can only be advertised in journals, by doctors or pharmaceutical representatives. Leo and Lacasse cite sertraline as an example of the effectiveness of the direct-to-consumer advertising campaign to promote the idea that SSRIs correct serotonin deficiency. Because of such advertising, sertraline has become the sixth most widely sold drug in the USA, with a sales volume of over three billion dollars in 2004.

Their work also reviews contrary evidence, as well as the lack of direct evidence for the chemical imbalance theory. One crucial point seems to be the limited control the FDA has over direct-to-consumer print, TV and internet advertising. Furthermore, even in the absence of scientific evidence, many claim that, as depression results from a serotonin deficit, it can be corrected by administering SSRIs. The examples reported relate to citalopram escitalopram, fluoxetine paroxetine and sertraline. The paper reports the arguments of authoritative scientists about the inconsistency of the theory (Lacasse and Leo 2005). Some of their arguments are reported below:

- Although it is often stated with great confidence that depressed people have a serotonin or norepinephrine deficiency, the evidence actually contradicts these claims (Valenstein 1998).
- Given the ubiquity of a neurotransmitter such as serotonin and the multiplicity of its functions, it is almost as meaningless to implicate it in depression as it is to implicate blood (Horgan 1999).
- Some have argued that depression may be due to a deficiency of norepinephrine or serotonin because the enhancement of noradrenergic or serotonergic neurotransmission improves the symptoms of depression. However, this is akin to saying that because a rash on one's arm improves with the use of a steroid cream, the rash must be due to a steroid deficiency (Delgado and Moreno 2000).
- Serotonin deficiency as an unconfirmed hypothesis, additional experience has not confirmed the monoamine depletion hypothesis (Dubvosky et al. 2003).
- No abnormality of serotonin in depression has ever been demonstrated (Healy 2004).

Two points should be mentioned here. The first concerns the treatment of anxiety disorders and the extraordinary rise of benzodiazepines. Even before SSRIs, benzodiazepines were used widely outside psychiatric institutions and they generated enormous profits. The initial enthusiasm of manufacturers and prescribers, justified by the irrefutable effectiveness of the drugs, played a key role in the debate around them. The fact that they could cause tolerance and both physical and psychological dependence was also a key factor. Judicious clinical use, however, can avoid the risk of dependence, which is relatively mild. Benzodiazepines in general also have only limited collateral and toxic effects. But when their patent expiry approached, which would have made them significantly less lucrative for their manufacturers, a large body of clinical evidence on the treatment of anxiety disorders with SSRI antidepressants (and other atypical compounds) began to grow. The clinical evidence highlights the problems of diagnosing depression and assessing the efficacy of antidepressants, but what is astonishing is the lack of reaction to the way SSRIs quickly replaced benzodiazepines in the treatment of anxiety disorders, despite the solid pharmacological and neurochemical evidence available.

The second point is that, while the debate about norepinephrine and serotonin's involvement in depression raged, a considerable body of sound biochemical pharmacological studies accumulated about anxiety. These showed that the action of benzodiazepines on anxiety was due to the potentiation of the effects of GABA,[12] an inhibitory neurotransmitter. The clinical efficacy of benzodiazepines was undisputed and could be traced to a specific neurochemical action mechanism. Benzodiazepines also worked effectively without any latency. It is therefore extremely surprising that SSRIs, which inhibit serotonin reuptake and whose mechanism had never been linked to anxiety and GABA before, suddenly replaced benzodiazepines as the primary treatment for anxiety disorders.

The properties of benzodiazepines and the use of antidepressants to treat anxiety are analysed thoroughly in Herzberg's book *Happy Pills in America. From Miltown to Prozac* (Herzberg 2009). The same process is related in detail in the book *All We Have to Fear: Psychiatry's Transformation of Natural Anxieties into Mental Disorders* by Horwitz and Wakefield. They previously published an important analysis of how sadness, a normal feeling and emotion, has been inappropriately transformed into a depressive disorder (Horwitz and Wakefield 2012).

Advances in neuroscience have helped us to understand the action mechanism of antidepressants, and a more in-depth investigation of the mechanisms of the brain may find new targets, helping with the development of new antidepressants. The monoamine theory has been followed by other, more sophisticated ones which take into account the molecular and cellular changes brought about by antidepressants, including brain reorganisation (Berton and Nestler 2006; Willner et al. 2013). An interesting example is brain neuroplasticity, namely the idea that the brain is able to reorganise itself in response to pharmacotherapy. In experiments that treated animals with antidepressants, it was found that neurone growth factors were released. BDNF[13] in particular caused a small but significant increase in the number of cells and synapses in a structure called the hippocampus. This theory would also account for the latency of antidepressant action. It should be noted, however, that the existing data on this was obtained using experimental models, and all current clinical data on the matter is of an indirect nature (BDNF levels in the blood or radiological images of the brain). As a result, definitive conclusions cannot be drawn about the neurobiological systems involved (Castrén and Rantamaki 2010).

A large amount of literature exists on the relationship between stress and depression. Starting with the initial, extensive and accurate observations of Paykel, a growing body of psychological literature suggests that difficulties adapting to life events may be one of the factors behind the onset of anxiety and depressive disorders (Hammen 2005; Paykel et al. 1969). However, developments in neuroscience have allowed us to gain an in-depth understanding of the neurobiological mechanisms common to stress and depression, and these show extremely complex scenarios (aan het Rot et al. 2009; Mahara et al. 2014; Manji et al. 2001; Nestler et al. 2002). The clinical significance of these studies is still far from clear (Hasler 2010); they also do not help with the problem of the chemical imbalance theory and the pharmacotherapy of depression.

These approaches highlight the complexity of the brain's mechanisms, and the difficulty of imagining methods of intervention that might be able to overcome the intrinsic resistance of such complex systems. This same complexity, which already makes it difficult to understand the action mechanisms of agents we know are effective, also makes it difficult to know whether new developments will work in the expected way.

Researchers with extensive experience reviewing the evolution of our understanding of the action mechanisms of antidepressants add that "the use of animal models has identified a number of novel targets some of which have been subjected to clinical trials in humans. However, monoamine antidepressants remain the best current medications and it may be some time before they are dislodged as the market leaders" (Slattery et al. 2004).

Two points need to be considered here. The first is how recent developments in biology and molecular genetics may affect depression and antidepressants. The second is to what extent SSRIs are actually, unlike tricyclics, devoid of adverse effects and safe for use. I will examine both in the following chapters.

Notes

1. Caused by the enzyme acetylcholinesterase.
2. For the purposes of this discussion, the neurotransmitters considered (norepinephrine, dopamine and serotonin) are called monoamines (to differentiate them from other amine derivatives that do not possess the neurotransmitter function). Based on their chemical structure, norepinephrine and dopamine are called catecholamines (produced in the neurones and originating from the amino acid phenylalanine); serotonin is called an indole compound, derived from the amino acid tryptophan.
3. Monoaminergic: mediated by the monoamines norepinephrine, dopamine and serotonin.
4. The transmission of a nerve impulse mediated by norepinephrine, dopamine and serotonin ends with the reuptake of the neurotransmitter.
5. The topic is significant both conceptually and in light of the growth of depression and its treatment using antidepressant drugs. There are many books on the subject, including: *The Myth of the Chemical Cure: A Critique of Psychiatric Drug Treatment* (Moncrieff 2007) and *Blaming the Brain: The Truth about Drugs and Mental Health* (Valenstein 1998).
6. The authors mentioned wrote this in connection to 3-methoxy-4-hydroxyphenylglycol (MHPG), considering it a possible metabolite from the degradation of norepinephrine.
7. Emphasis added by the author.
8. "Equivalent" refers to a product whose active molecule has an expired patent and is therefore cheaper.
9. Meaning outside those specified by regulatory body approval.
10. The nature and extent of these effects has already been discussed in previous chapters.
11. The issue is significant and has been widely debated in scientific literature. Copious references can be found on the David Healy website (http://davidhealy.org/).
12. γ-Aminobutyric acid, the main inhibitory neurotransmitter in the central nervous system.
13. BDNF: brain-derived neurotrophic factor.

References

aan het Rot, M., Mathew, S. J., & Charney, D. S. (2009). Neurobiological mechanisms in major depressive disorder. *Canadian Medical Association Journal, 180*(3), 305–313.

Angell, M. (2004). *The truth about the drug companies: How they deceive us and what to do about it.* New York: Random House.

Baughman, F. (2006). There is no such thing as a psychiatric disorder/ disease/ chemical imbalance. *PLoS Med, 3*(7), e318.

Baumeister, A. A., Hawkins, M. F., & Uzelac, S. M. (2003). The myth of the reserpine—Induced depression: Role in the historical development of the monoamine hypothesis. *Journal of the History of Neurosciences, 12*(2), 207–220.

Beers, M. H., & Passman, L. J. (1990). Antihypertensive medications and depression. *Drugs, 40*(6), 792–799.

Belmaker, R. H., & Agam, G. (2008). Major depressive disorder. *New England Journal of Medicine, 358*, 55–68.

Benarroch, E. E. (2009). The locus ceruleus norepinephrine system: Functional organization and potential clinical significance. *Neurology, 73*(20), 1699–1704.

Bennett, M. R. (1998). Monoaminergic synapses and schizophrenia: 45 years of neuroleptics. *Journal of Psychopharmacology, 12*, 289–304.

Berger, M., Gray, J. A., & Roth, B. L. (2009). The expanded biology of serotonin. *Annual Reviews of Medicine, 60*, 355–366.

Berton, O., & Nestler, E. J. (2006). New approaches to antidepressant drug discovery: Beyond monoamines. *Nature Reviews Neuroscience, 7*, 137–151.

Bowers, M. B. (1974). Lumbar CSF 5-hydroxyindoleacetic acid and homovanillic acid in affective syndromes. *Journal of Nervous and Mental Diseases, 158*(5), 325–330.

Bowers, M. B., Heninger, G. R., & Gerbode, F. (1969). Cerebrospinal fluid 5-hydroxyindoleactiic acid and homovanillic acid in psychiatric patients. *International Journal of Neuropharmacology, 8*(3), 255–262.

Brink, C. B., Harvey, B. H., & Brand, L. (2006). Tianeptine: A novel atypical antidepressant that may provide new insights into the biomolecular basis of depression. *Recent Patents on CNS Drug Discovery, 1*(1), 29–41.

Castrén, E. (2005). Is mood chemistry? *Nature Reviews Neurosciences, 6*(3), 241–246.

Castrén, E., & Rantamaki, T. (2010). The role of BDNF and its receptors in depression and antidepressant drug action: Reactivation of developmental plasticity. *Developmental Neurobiology, 70*(5), 289–297.

Cipriani, A., Furukawa, T. A., Salanti, G., Geddes, J. R., Higgins, J. P., Churchill, R., Watanabe, N., Nakagawa, A., Omori, I. M., McGuire, H., Tansella, M., & Barbui, C. (2009). Comparative efficacy and acceptability of 12 new-generation antidepressants: A multiple-treatments meta analysis. *Lancet, 73*, 746–758.

Davies, D. L., & Shepherd, M. (1955). Reserpine in the treatment of anxious and depressed patients. *Lancet, 269*(6881), 117–120.

Delgado, P., & Moreno, F. (2000). Role of norepinephrine in depression. *Journal of Clinical Psychiatry, 61*(1), 5–12.

Delgado, P. L., Price, L. H., Miller, H. L., Salomon, R. M., Aghajanian, G. K., Heninger, G. R., & Charney D. S. (1994). Serotonin and the neurobiology of depression. Effects of tryptophan depletion in drug-free depressed patients. *Archives of General Psychiatry, 51*(11), 865–874.

Dubvosky, S., Davies, R., & Dubvosky, A. (2003). Mood disorders. In R. Yudofsky & S. Hales (Eds.), *The american psychiatric textbook of clinical psychiatry* (pp. 439–542). Washington, DC: American Psychiatric Press.

Eyding, D., Lelgemann, M., Grouven, U., Härter, M., Kromp, M., Kaiser, T., Kerekes, M. F., Gerken, M., & Wieseler, B. (2010). Reboxetine for acute treatment of major depression: Systematic review and meta-analysis of published and unpublished placebo and selective serotonin reuptake inhibitor controlled trials. *British Medical Journal, 341*, c4737.

Glowinski, J., & Axelrod, J. (1964). Inhibition of uptake of tritiated-noradrenaline in the intact rat brain by imipramine and structurally related compounds. *Nature, 204*, 1318–1319.

Hammen, C. (2005). Stress and depression. *Annual Review of Clinical Psychology, 1*, 293–319.

Hasler, G. (2010). Pathophysiology of depression: Do we have any solid evidence of interest to clinicians? *World Psychiatry, 9*, 155–161.

Healy, D. (2004). *Let them eat prozac: The unhealthy relationship between the pharmaceutical companies and depression.* New York: New York University Press.

Herzberg, D. (2009). *Happy pills in America: From miltown to prozac.* Baltimore: John Hopkins University Press.

Horgan, J. (1999). *The undiscovered mind: How the human brain defies replication, medication, and explanation.* New York: Free Press.

Horwitz, A. V., & Wakefield, J. C. (2012). *All we have to fear: Psychiatry's transformation of natural anxieties into mental disorders.* Oxford: Oxford University Press.

Humble, M. (2000). Noradrenaline and serotonin reuptake inhibition as clinical principles: A review of antidepressant efficacy. *Acta Psychiatrica Scandinavica, 101*(Suppl. 402), 28–36.

Ig Nobel Prize. (2000). *May we recommend—The science of romantic love.* http://www.improb.com/news/2002/feb/romantic.html. Accessed 15 April, 2015.

Karch, S. B. (1999). Cocaine: History, use, abuse. *Journal of the Royal Society of Medicine, 92*(8), 393–397.

Lacasse, J. R., & Leo, J. (2005). Serotonin and depression: A disconnect between the advertisements and the scientific literature. *PLoS Med, 2*(12), e392.

Lahti, R. A., & Maickel, R. P. (1971). The tricyclic antidepressants-inhibition of norepinephrine uptake as related to potentiation of norepinephrine and clinical efficacy. *Biochemical Pharmacology, 20*(2), 482–486.

Leo, J., & Lacasse, J. R. (2008). The media and the chemical imbalance theory of depression. *Society, 45*(1), 35–45.

Leucht, C., Huhn, M., & Leucht, S. (2012). Amitriptyline versus placebo for major depressive disorder. *Cochrane Database of Systematic Reviews*, (2). doi: 10.1002/14651858.

López-Muñoz, F., & Alamo, C. (2009a). Historical evolution of the neurotransmission concept. *Journal of Neural Transmission, 116*(5), 515–533.

López-Muñoz, F., & Alamo, C. (2009b). Monoaminergic neurotransmission: The history of the discovery of antidepressants from 1950s until today. *Current Pharmaceutical Design, 15*(14), 1563–1586.

Maas, J. W., Koslow, S. H., Katz, M. M., et al. (1984). Pretreatment neurotransmitter metabolite levels and response to tricyclic antidepressant drugs. *American Journal of Psychiatry, 14*(10), 1159–1171.

Magarian, G. J. (1991). Reserpine: A relic from the past or a neglected drug of the present for achieving cost containment in treating hypertension? *Journal of General and Internal Medicine, 6*(6), 561–572.

Mahara, I., Bambicoc, F. C., Mechawara, N., & Nobrega, J. N. (2014). Stress, serotonin, and hippocampal neurogenesis in relation to depression and antidepressant effects. *Neuroscience and Biobehavioral Reviews, 38,* 173–192.

Manji, H. K., Drevets, W. C., & Charney, D. S. (2001). The cellular neurobiology of depression. *Nature Medicine, 7,* 541–547.

Marazziti, D., Akiskal, H. S., Rossi, A., & Cassano, G. B. (1999). Alteration of the platelet serotonin transporter in romantic love. *Psychological Medicine, 29*(3), 741–745.

McEwen, B. S., Chattarji, S., Diamond, D. M., Jay, T. M., Reagan, L. P., Svenningsson, P., & Fuchs, E. (2010). The neurobiological properties of tianeptine (Stablon): From monoamine hypothesis to glutamatergic modulation. *Molecular Psychiatry, 15*(3), 237–249.

McGeer, P. L., & McGeer, E. G. (1980). Chemistry of mood and emotion. *Annual Reviews of Psychology, 31,* 273–307.

Mendels, J., & Frazer, A. (1974). Brain biogenic amine depletion and mood. *Archives of Genral Psychiatry, 30*(4), 447–451.

Moncrieff, J. (2007). *The myth of the chemical cure: A critique of psychiatric drug treatment.* Basingstoke: Palgrave Macmillan.

Mulinari, S. (2012). Monoamine theories of depression: Historical impact on biomedical research. *Journal of the History of the Neurosciences: Basic and Clinical Perspectives, 21*(4), 366–392.

Nestler, E.J., Barrot, M., DiLeone, R.J. Eisch, A. J., Gold, S. J., & Monteggia, L. M. (2002). Neurobiology of Depression. *Neuron, 34*(1): 13–25.

Nobel Prize in Physiology and Medicine. (1936).http://www.nobelprize.org/nobel_prizes/medicine/laureates/1936/. Accessed 3 February, 2015.

Nobel Prize in Physiology and Medicine. (1970). http://www.nobelprize.org/nobel_prizes/medicine/laureates/1970/. Accessed March 3, 2015.

Papeschi, R., & McClure, D. J. (1971). Homovanillic and 5-hydroxyindoleacetic acid in cerebrospinal fluid of depressed patients. *Archives of General Psychiatry, 25*(4), 354–358.

Paykel, E. S., Myers, J. K., Dienelt, M. N., Klerman, G. L., Lindenthal, J. J., & Pepper, M. P. (1969). Life events and depression: A controlled study. *Archives of General Psychiatry, 21*(6), 753–760.

Racagni, G., & Popoli, M. (2008). Cellular and molecular mechanisms in the long-term action of antidepressants. *Dialogues in Clinical Neurosciences, 10*(4), 385–400.

Rasmussen, R. (2008). A quantitative and qualitative retrospective with implications for the present America's first amphetamine epidemic 1929–1971. *American Journal of Public Health, 98*(6), 974–985.

Ravindran, A. V., & da Silva, T. L. (2013). Review complementary and alternative therapies as add-onto pharmacotherapy for mood and anxiety disorders: A systematic review. *Journal of Affective Disorders, 150*(3), 707–719.

Ross, S. B., & Renyi, A. L. (1967). Inhibition of the uptake of tritiated catecholamines by antidepressant and related agents. *European Journal of Pharmacology, 2*(3), 181–186.

Ross, S. B., & Renyi, A. L. (1969). Inhibition of the uptake of tritiated 5-hydroxytryptamine in brain tissue. *European Journal of Pharmacology, 7*(3), 270–277.

Rothman, R. B., Baumann, M. H., Dersch, C. M., Romero, D. V., Rice, K. C., Carroll, F. I., & Partilla J. S. (2001). Amphetamine-type central nervous system stimulants release norepinephrine more potently than they release dopamine and serotonin. *Synapse, 39*(1), 32–41.

Ruetsch, Y. A., Boni, T., & Borgeat, A. (2001). From cocaine to ropivacaine: The history of local anesthetic drugs. *Current Topics in Medicinal Chemistry, 1*(3), 175–182.

Schildkraut, J. J. (1965). The catecholamine hypothesis of affective disorders: A review of the supportive evidence. *American Journal of Psychiatry, 122*(5), 509–522.

Slattery, D. A., Hudson, A. L., & Nutt, D. J. (2004). Invited review: The evolution of antidepressant mechanisms. *Fundamental & Clinical Pharmacology, 18*(1), 1–21.

Sulzer, D., Sonders, M. S., Poulsen, N. W., & Galli, A. (2005). Mechanisms of neurotransmitter release by amphetamines: A review. *Progress in Neurobiology, 75*(6), 406–433.

Svensson, T. H. (2000). Brain noradrenaline and the mechanisms of action of antidepressant drugs. *Acta Psychiatrica Scandinavica, 402*(Suppl. 2000) 18–27.

Valenstein, E. S. (1998). *Blaming the brain: The truth about drugs and mental health*. New York: Free Press.

Willner, P., Scheel-Krügerb, J., & Belzung, C. (2013). The neurobiology of depression and antidepressant action. *Neuroscience and Biobehavioral Reviews, 37*(10 Part 1): 2331–2371.

Wong, D. T., Perry, K. W., & Bymaster, F. P. (2005). The discovery of fluoxetine hydrochloride (Prozac). *Nature Reviews Drug Discovery, 4,* 764–774.

Wrobel, S. (2007). Science, serotonin, and sadness: The biology of antidepressants. *The FASEB Journal, 21*(13), 3404–3417.

Young, L. J. (2009). Being human: Love: Neuroscience reveals all. *Nature, 457*(7226), 148. doi:10.1038/457148a.

10

Written in the Genes

Clarke's Third Law: Any sufficiently advanced technology is indistinguishable from magic.
Arthur C. Clarke

So far the evidence on the action mechanisms of antidepressants had been biochemical in nature. Much of it was gathered in the period immediately after the Second World War, when there were extraordinary advances in our basic and clinical knowledge of the nervous system. During this period neurotransmitters were discovered, and we developed an understanding of the electrochemical mechanisms of neurotransmission. Psychotropic drugs such as tranquilisers, antipsychotics, antidepressants and antimanic drugs were also developed in this period, which made pharmacotherapeutic treatments for psychiatric illnesses possible for the first time. As shown in the previous chapter, this coincided with the essentially unsuccessful attempt to reduce mental disorders to alterations in the brain's chemistry, and to reduce the action of psychotropic drugs to the correction of these alterations.

The experimental studies performed in this field could be defined as essentially phenotypic: examinations of the chemical nature of

© The Author(s) 2017
T. Giraldi, *Unhappiness, Sadness and 'Depression'*,
DOI 10.1007/978-3-319-57657-2_10

cellular components (an area traditionally associated with biochemistry). Studies in this field have covered both functions and reciprocal interactions (more often associated with physiology studies), as well as changes to their functions caused by drugs and other substances (more often associated with pharmacology).

The following years saw even more extraordinary advances in molecular biology, and soon we began to develop an understanding of DNA and the chemically coded genetic heritage it contains. DNA is essentially comprised of a sequence of purine[1] and pyrimidine[2] bases, and each human cell has a double strand of DNA at its core, which contains over six billion bases: it would be a total of about three metres long if it was completely unrolled. DNA is contained in structures called genes, located in 46 chromosomes in the nuclei of cells. The Human Genome Project set out to map the entire sequence of human DNA bases, and its aim was to identify their precise nature and position in the DNA. It ended in 2000 and estimated the total number of human genes at between 20,000 and 25,000[3] (Lander 2001; Venter et al. 2001; Venter 2007).

The genes encode all the characteristics of the phenotype, which differentiate one person from another and which are passed on to people's descendants as a genotype: traits such as sex, hair and eye colour, height, weight and so forth. Molecular biology has been able to combine the techniques of biology and molecular genetics into an approach called genomics, which investigates individual characteristics. Individual differences have been traced back to the existence of genetic polymorphisms which arose from: different numbers of active gene copies, mutations caused by the replacement of individual bases in the DNA strand—called SNP[4]—and the insertion or deletion of base sequences called LPR[5] and VNTR .[6]

A key question for genomics is whether, amid all the individual differences, there is a cause or concause of illnesses, written in our genome. Another important question is whether medicinal drugs cause different responses depending on the genetic-molecular background of the patient. These are complex issues that require an extended discussion, but that is beyond the remit of this work. Here I will limit myself to considering these questions in relation to depression and antidepressants.

A 2003 paper by the English psychiatrist Caspi and his collaborators, published in the American magazine *Science*, attracted considerable
attention (Caspi et al. 2003). The group worked on the hypothesis that
there is a genetic polymorphism involving the synaptic transporter of
serotonin. This polymorphism occurs, the study suggested, in a DNA
region called the promoter, which regulates the function of the gene,
and can exist in two variations: "short" ("s") or "long" ("l"), depending
on whether it contains a sequence of 44 base pairs. The short variation
corresponds to a carrier protein with reduced functionality.[7] There are
two copies of all our genes in the nuclei of our cells, each originating
from one parent. As far as the serotonin transporter gene is concerned,
25% of all people will have the "s/s" genotype, 50% will have the "s/l"
genotype, and 25% will have the "l/l" genotype, depending on the variants they have inherited from their parents. The functionality of the
serotonin transporter in each individual is thus low ("s/s"), intermediate
("s/l") or high ("l/l")[8] (Lesch et al. 1996).

This was followed by a large number of studies of 5-HTTLPR. They
were carried out to determine serotonin's involvement in a variety of
healthy and unhealthy brain functions, and also to determine whether
the serotonin transporter is one of the significant factors in neurotransmission. 5-HTTLPR thus became the most investigated genetic variant
in psychiatry, psychology and neuroscience (Caspi et al. 2010). It has
been associated with a variety of conditions such as neuroticism (Gonda
et al. 2009) and has been dubbed the "Woody Allen gene" (Kramer
2003). It has also been associated with depression, anxiety (Middeldorp
et al. 2007), post-traumatic stress disorders (PTSD) (Gressier et al.
2013), obsessive compulsive disorders (OCD) (Hu et al. 2006), suicidal
tendencies (Anguelova et al. 2003) and even wellbeing and happiness
(De Neve 2011).

The starting point for Caspi's study was that people who had experienced stressful life events, threats, loss, humiliation or defeats often
succumbed to depression. To investigate why this did not occur in all
people and to the same extent, Caspi's team gathered information from
1037 young New Zealanders aged 21–26. The information covered a
range of stressful life events relating to employment, economic, housing
and family problems. The young people were investigated to see if they

had been diagnosed with major depression in the preceding year. The subjects were also classified by the genotype of their serotonin transporter 5-HTTLPR.

The results showed that individuals with one or two copies of the "short" gene variant ("s/s" and "s/l") had more pronounced symptoms of depression, diagnosable depression and suicidal risk in relation to the number of stressful life events they had experienced. The authors therefore postulated the existence of a gene–environment interaction,[9] whereby an individual response to environmental influences could be accentuated by an unfavourable genetic constitution. This is extremely interesting because, if true, it would overcome the difficulty of tracing the onset of depression to *either* stressful life events *or* genetic polymorphism (5-HTTLPR "s/s" or "s/l"). It would also suggest that it is the *combination* of the two factors that leads to a greater probability of more severe depressive tendencies (Caspi et al. 2003, 2010).

As with other areas, the growing number of studies available has made it possible to use meta-analysis. In 2009, meta-analysis by Munafò and his collaborators concluded that the available data was "compatible with chance findings" (Munafò et al. 2009). In the same year, Risch's meta-analysis was just as negative, concluding that there "was no evidence that the serotonin transporter genotype alone or in interaction with stressful life events is associated with an elevated risk of depression…in both sexes" (Risch et al. 2009). In 2011, the inclusion of a wider number of publications led to the opposite conclusion, namely that there was "strong evidence that 5-HTTLPR moderates the relationship between stress and depression in the studies published to date" (Karg et al. 2011).

Despite the controversy surrounding the published meta-analysis, some interesting points did emerge. In attempts to correlate the vulnerable "short" variant (the genotype) with the onset of depression (the phenotype), the latter remains labile because it consists of a myriad of symptoms rather than a small number of incontrovertible somatic symptoms. In addition, the overall variability of the individual's propensity to develop a depressive disorder—the part of the phenomenon accounted for by 5-HTTLPR—is very limited (Blakely and Veenstra-VanderWeele 2011).

The characteristics of individual genotypes were examined in about half the subjects in the STAR*D study, and a number of polymorphisms were considered, including the serotonin transporter (Laje et al. 2009). Overall, they found there was a lack of correlation between the polymorphisms and the response to citalopram (Garriock and Hamilton 2009). The results of the study are very interesting and indicate limited associations with suicidal behaviour and depression-related personality traits, although they are not significantly associated with major depressive disorder itself (Levinson 2006).

In addition to the studies into the onset of depression, genetic molecular approaches have also been used to examine the response to antidepressant treatment. These studies fall under the new research field of pharmacogenetics and relate to the possible individualisation of pharmacotherapy (Evans and Johnson 2001; Evans and McLeod 2003). The clinical pharmacokinetics of antidepressants have also been investigated: this essentially involves the study of the drug concentration present in the body during treatment. These studies delivered apparently relevant results, but unlike the results for other pharmacotherapeutic treatments—such as those for manic depressive psychosis[10]—they have not yet been introduced into clinical practice (Hiemke and Härtter 2000; Sjöqvist and Bertilsson 1984; Van Brunt 1983). The pharmacogenetic approaches applied to pharmacokinetics are also equally relevant, but they have not yet been introduced into clinical practice either (Weinshilboum 2003; Narasimhan and Lohoff 2012).

There are clear reasons for the extensive interest in the role of the serotonin transporter gene polymorphism 5-HTTLPR in relation to the effects of antidepressants (pharmacodynamics). According to the serotonin deficit theory, selective serotonin reuptake inhibitors (SSRIs) should increase the synaptic concentration of the neurotransmitter, and they should be made more effective if polymorphism strengthens the action of the transporter.

A great number of studies were published in this area, which made meta-analysis possible. This indicated that "in Caucasians, 5-HTTLPR may be a predictor of antidepressant response and remission, while in Asians it does not appear to play a major role"[11] (Porcelli et al. 2012). A study that reported the results of randomised controlled trials on the pharmacogenetics of SSRIs concluded that "it is unlikely that the 5-HTTLPR polymorphism alone will be clinically useful in predicting response to antidepressants in depressed patients" (Lewis et al. 2011). The article was preceded by an editorial that stated, "there probably is a real, if small, effect of 5-HTTLPR on response to both serotonin reuptake inhibitors and environmental adversity" (McGuffin et al. 2011).

Although studies into the connection between 5-HTTLPR and antidepressant responses produced limited results, a series of studies called the Genome-Wide Association Scan (GWAS) were conducted. These studies examined large parts of the DNA of a group of subjects, looking for polymorphism relating to certain conditions (Malhotra 2010). So far they have provided results of no or little significance and limited replicability. In fact, the results are often contradictory, and the risk factors identified are of extremely limited size and unlikely to have clinical application (Laje and McMahon 2011). The GWAS studies have been extended to integrate neuroimaging data obtained through modern techniques, but even in this case the results are of an experimental nature and have uncertain clinical applications (Savitz and Drevets 2009).

Returning to the subject of the serotonin transporter, the connection of 5-HTTLPR with the onset of depression seems uncertain, and its usefulness for determining the magnitude of the response to SSRI antidepressants seems limited. The inconclusiveness of the results is partly due to the complexity of depression from a psychological neurobiological and genetic-molecular perspective. It is also partially due to the inadequate definition of phenotypic traits in the depressed (Blakely and Veenstra-VanderWeele 2011). This is also why the effects of antidepressants are almost indistinguishable from placebos in mild and moderate cases of depression. This might seem at odds with the data on the pharmacogenetics of antidepressants, which shows a significant if modest improvement in subjects carrying the "l" variant of 5-HTTLPR.

While examining this subject, it may be useful to consider the results of an impeccably designed study carried out using both neuroimaging and genetic-molecular analysis. The study set out to examine the brain's response to exposure to a socially stressful situation (public speaking) as a model of social anxiety disorder. The experimental subjects were geno-typed for 5-HTTLPR and treated with a placebo. The study found that the placebo caused reduced stress activity in the amygdala, a part of the brain vital for emotional processing, but that this only occurred in sub-jects who carried the "l/l" variant of 5-HTTLPR (Furmark et al. 2008). The placebo effect therefore depends on 5-HTTLPR, and it is impor-tant to bear this in mind when considering the similar effects of place-bos and antidepressants on mild to moderate depression.

The pharmacogenetics of the relationship between SSRIs and the polymorphism 5-HTTLPR are consistent with the general hypothesis about their action mechanism. Subjects with "long" ("l") variants—causing higher functional activity—respond better to SSRIs, which inhibit serotonin reuptake, causing a higher concentration of seroto-nin in the synapses, which corrects the initial deficit. The results with the "short" ("s") variant—causing lower functional reuptake activity—remain mixed, and the variant has often been ignored in corresponding literature. Overall, however, "s" subjects are more prone to depression when there is a higher concentration of serotonin in the synapses—the very condition caused by SSRIs. This continues to contradict the theory that mood disorders are caused by monoamine deficit.

Notes

1. Adenine and guanine.
2. Thymine and cytosine.
3. The fact that it is an estimate is startling, but this derives from the tech-niques used, which have not directly examined all three billion DNA bases but only those from regions of particular interest.
4. SNP: Single-Nucleotide Polymorphism.
5. LPR: Length-Restricted Polymorphism—base sequences of diverging length.
6. VNTR: Variable Number of Tandem Repeats—the presence of repeat sequence bases.

7. This polymorphism is called Length-Restricted Polymorphism and concerns the transporter (T) of serotonin (5-HT), called 5-HTTLPR.
8. In the work cited by Lesch, the serotonin transporter function is assessed by the serotonin reuptake in in vitro human cells.
9. Gene × Environment (G × E).
10. For example, the lithium salts used to cure bipolar disorder are administered in doses determined after monitoring the concentration of lithium in the blood.
11. It should be noted that the magnitude of this phenomenon is relatively limited: the genetic polymorphism taken into consideration causes a difference of a factor of circa 1.5.

References

Anguelova, M., Benkelfat, C., & Turecki, G. (2003). A systematic review of association studies investigating genes coding for serotonin receptors and the serotonin transporter: II. Suicidal behavior. *Molecular Psychiatry, 8,* 646–653.

Blakely, R. D., & Veenstra-VanderWeele, J. (2011). Genetic Indeterminism, the 5-HTTLPR, and the paths forward. *Neuropsychiatric Genetics, Archives of General Psychiatry, 68*(5), 457–458.

Caspi, A., Hariri, A. R., Holmes, A., Uher, R., & Moffitt, T. E. (2010). Genetic sensitivity to the environment: The case of the serotonin transporter gene and its implications for studying complex diseases and traits. *American Journal of Psychiatry, 167*(5), 509–527.

Caspi, A., Sugden, K., Moffitt, T. E., Taylor, A., Craig, I. W., Harrington, H., McClay, J., Mill, J., Martin, J., Braithwaite, A., & Poulton, R. (2003). Influence of life stress on depression: Moderation by a polymorphism in the 5-HTT gene. *Science, 301*(5631), 386–389.

De Neve, J. E. (2011). Functional polymorphism (5-HTTLPR) in the serotonin transporter gene is associated with subjective well-being: Evidence from a US nationally representative sample. *Journal of Human Genetics, 56*(6), 456–459.

Evans, W. E., & Johnson, J. A. (2001). Pharmacogenomics: The inherited basis for interindividual differences in drug response. *Annual Reviews of Genomics and Human Genetics, 2,* 9–39.

Evans, W. E., & McLeod, H. L. (2003). Review article. Drug therapy. Pharmacogenomics—Drug disposition, drug targets, and side effects. *New England Journal of Medicine, 348*(6), 538–549.

Furmark, T., Appel, L., Henningsson, S., Åhs, F., Faria, V., Linnman, C., Pissiota, A., Frans, O., Bani, M., Bettica, P., Pich, E. M., Jacobsson, E., Wahlstedt, K., Oreland. L., Långström, B., Eriksson, E., & Fredrikson, M. (2008). A link between serotonin-related gene polymorphisms, amygdala activity, and placebo-induced relief from social anxiety. *The Journal of Neuroscience, 28*(49), 13066–13074.

Garriock, H. A., & Hamilton, S. P. (2009). Genetic studies of drug response and side effects in the STAR*D study, part 1. *Journal of Clinical Psychiatry, 70*(8), 1186–1187.

Gonda, X., Fountoulakis, K. N., Juhasz, G., Rihmer, Z., Judit Lazary, J., Laszik, A., Hagop, S., Akiskal, H. S., & Bagdy, G. (2009). Association of the s allele of the 5-HTTLPR with neuroticism-related traits and temperaments in a psychiatrically healthy population. *European Archives of Psychiatry and Clinical Neurological Sciences, 259*(2), 106–113.

Gressier, F., Calati, R., Balestri, M., Marsano, A., Alberti, S., Antypa, N., & Serretti, A. (2013). The 5-HTTLPR polymorphism and posttraumatic stress disorder: A meta-Analysis. *Journal of Traumatic Stress, 26*(6), 645–653.

Hiemke, C., & Härtter, S. (2000). Pharmacokinetics of selective serotonin reuptake inhibitors. *Pharmacology & Therapeutics, 85*(1), 11–28.

Hu, X. Z., Lipsky, R. H., Zhu, G., Akhtar, L. A., Taubman, J., Greenberg, B. D., Xu, K., Arnold, P. D., Richter, M. A., Kennedy, J. L., Murphy, D. L., & Goldman, D. (2006). Serotonin transporter promoter gain-of-function genotypes are linked to obsessive-compulsive disorder. *The American Journal of Human Genetics, 78*(5), 815–826.

Karg, K., Burmeister, M., Shedden, K., & Sen, S. (2011). The serotonin transporter promoter variant (5-HTTLPR), stress, and depression. Meta-analysis revisited. Evidence of genetic moderation. *Archives of General Psychiatry, 68*(5), 444–454.

Kramer, P. D. (2003). Tapping the mood gene. *The New York Times*. http://www.nytimes.com/2003/07/26/opinion/tapping-the-mood-gene.html. Accessed 24 Feb 2015.

Laje, G., & McMahon, F. J. (2011). Genome-wide association studies of antidepressant outcome: A brief review. *Progress in Neuro-Psychopharmacology and Biological Psychiatry, 35*(7), 1553–1557.

Laje, G., Perlis, R. H., Rush, A. J., & McMahon, F. J. (2009). Pharmacogenetics studies in STAR*D: Strengths, limitations, and results. *Psychiatric Services, 60*(11), 1446–1457.

Lander, E. S. (2001). Human genome. *Nature, 409*(6822), 860–921.

Lesch, K. P., Bengel, D., Heils, A., Sabol, S. Z., Greenberg, B. D., Petri, S., Benjamin, J., Müller, C. R., Hamer, D. H., & Murphy, D. L. (1996). Association of anxiety-related traits with a polymorphism in the serotonin transporter gene regulatory region. *Science, 274*(5292), 1527–1531.

Levinson, D. F. (2006). The genetics of depression: A review. *Biological Psychiatry, 60*(2), 84–92.

Lewis, G., Mulligan, J., Wiles, N., Cowen, P., Craddock, N., Ikeda, M., Grozeva, D., Mason, V., Nutt, D., Sharp, D., Tallon, D., Thomas, L., O'Donovan, M. C., & Peters, T. J. (2011). Polymorphism of the 5-HT transporter and response to antidepressants: Randomised controlled trial. *British Journal of Psychiatry, 198*(6), 464–471.

Malhotra, A. K. (2010). The pharmacogenetics of depression: Enter the GWAS. *American Journal of Psychiatry, 167*(5), 493–495.

McGuffin, P., Alsabban, S., & Uher, R. (2011). The truth about genetic variation in the serotonin transporter gene and response to stress and medication. *British Journal of Psychiatry, 198*(6), 424–427.

Middeldorp, C. M., de Geus, E. J. C., Beem, A. E., Lakenberg, N., Hottenga, J. J., Slagboom, P. E., & Boomsma, D. I. (2007). Family based association analyses between the serotonin transporter gene polymorphism (5-HTTLPR) and neuroticism, anxiety and depression. *Behavioural Genetics, 37*(2), 294–301.

Munafò, M. R., Durrant, C., Lewis, G., & Flint, J. (2009). Gene × Environment interactions at the serotonin transporter locus. *Biological Psychiatry, 65*(3), 211–219.

Narasimhan, S., & Lohoff, F. W. (2012). Pharmacogenetics of antidepressant drugs: Current clinical practice and future directions. *Pharmacogenomics, 13*(4), 441–464.

Porcelli, S., Fabbri, C., & Serretti, A. (2012). Meta-analysis of serotonin transporter gene promoter polymorphism (5-HTTLPR) association with antidepressant efficacy. *European Neuropsychopharmacology, 22*(4), 239–258.

Risch, N., Herrell, R., Lehner, T., Liang, K. Y., Eaves, L., Hoh, J., Griem, A., Kovacs, M., Ott, J., & Merikangas, K. R. (2009). Interaction between the serotonin transporter gene (5-HTTLPR), stressful life events, and risk of depression: A meta-analysis. *The Journal of American Medical Association, 301*(23), 2462–2471.

Savitz, J. B., & Drevets, W. C. (2009). Imaging phenotypes of major depressive disorder: Genetic correlates. *Neuroscience, 164*(1), 300–330.

Sjöqvist, F., & Bertilsson, L. (1984). Clinical pharmacology of antidepressant drugs: Pharmacogenetics. *Advances in Biochemical Psychopharmacology, 39,* 359–372.

Van Brunt, N. (1983). The clinical utility of tricyclic antidepressant blood levels: A review of the literature. *Therapeutic Drug Monitoring, 5*(1), 1–10.

Venter, J. C. (2007). *A life decoded: My genome: My life.* London: Allen Lane Science.

Venter, J. C., Adams M. D., Myers E. W., Li, P. W., Mural, R. J., Sutton, G. G. et al. (2001). The sequence of the human genome. *Science, 16*(291 (5507)), 1304–1351.

Weinshilboum, R. (2003). Inheritance and drug response. *New England Journal of Medicine, 348,* 529–537.

11

The Safety of Antidepressants

One of the first duties of the physician is to educate the masses
not to take medicine.
William Osler

When substances such as the antituberculosis agents isoniazid and iproniazid and the tricyclic imipramine were shown to have antidepressant
actions, they made it possible to treat depressive mood disorders effectively for the first time. Until the extraordinary advances of the 1950
and 1960 there was no way to counteract the effects of major depression, but, fortunately, this condition had been extremely limited until
then. Those who suffered from it were taken into psychiatric care, which
was provided by mental health institutions or private clinics for the
wealthy. Some suffering from mild depression—presumably non-psy-
chotic and often provoked by life events—were deemed to be suffering
from neurotic disorders and could be treated using psychoanalysis and
psychotherapy. But this category was subsequently struck from the language of biological psychiatry and the Diagnostic and Statistical Manual
of Mental Disorders (DSM). In light of all this, the creation of effective pharmacotherapeutic treatments was an extraordinary development

© The Author(s) 2017   **153**
T. Giraldi, *Unhappiness, Sadness and 'Depression',*
DOI 10.1007/978-3-319-57657-2_11

indeed. New pharmacotherapeutic treatments could completely revitalise patients who would otherwise have been condemned to suffer the full range of depression symptoms.

During this period, serious depression was referred to as either endogenous or vital depression. The former originated from within the sufferer and could not be traced to life events. The latter was characterised by serious difficulty in both organising and deriving pleasure from one's own activities. Fortunately, more serious forms of depression were comparatively rare, and soon it became possible to treat them effectively with antidepressants. Sometimes it was possible to use shorter treatments, which could be interrupted when the patient overcame a depressive episode.

Although tricyclic antidepressants were effective, they also caused pronounced and adverse side effects. But in severe cases it's not surprising that the effectiveness of the treatment was considered to be worth the adverse effects, and fortunately, although tricyclic antidepressants have a similar chemical structure to antipsychotics—and have many adverse effects in common—they do not cause the same serious movement disorders (Freedman 2003; Mann 2005).

Monoamine oxidase inhibitors were another matter. They had very different possible side effects, such as damage to the peripheral nervous system and liver, which were sometimes catastrophic in people more susceptible to their toxic effects. What people then saw as idiosyncrasy, we now understand was caused by a genetic polymorphism that made certain individuals much less able to metabolise and inactivate drugs. It also meant those individuals were much more likely to have higher plasma concentrations, causing greater toxicity after conventional drug doses (Meyer 2000). Because of their action mechanism, monoamine oxidase inhibitors also have long-term effects, which means they are more likely to interact with other drugs, with harmful effects. Unsurprisingly, they have been practically abandoned, except for a few newer molecules with better efficacy and safety profiles (Shulman et al. 2013).

There has been a rapid increase in the volume of selective serotonin reuptake inhibitors (SSRIs) prescribed since fluoxetine entered the market, and this is essentially because the general view is that they are more effective and have fewer negative side effects than tricyclic antidepressants. Their effectiveness has already been discussed in the previous chapter; this chapter will focus on their adverse side effects. Some are intrinsically linked to the action mechanism. Others, however, were not anticipated and were instead discovered in clinical practice and observation after the drugs were authorised.

The belief that SSRI antidepressants are well tolerated and better than tricyclic antidepressants is based on their more selective action mechanism. SSRIs work by inhibiting the reuptake of serotonin, which allows them to avoid the side effects caused by inhibiting the reuptake of norepinephrine. As a result, the principal adverse effect is serotonin syndrome, a condition caused by an excessive SSRI dose, or the combination of SSRIs with other treatments that stimulate serotonin release. Serotonin syndrome varies in severity depending on the dosage received, and it manifests itself with restless movement, tremors, mental changes, seizures and high temperatures. It can even be fatal in the most severe cases (Boyer and Shannon 2005).

Initial studies of tricyclic antidepressants' action mechanisms suggested that they did not just inhibit the reuptake of serotonin and norepinephrine in the presynaptic nerve, but also inhibited the post-synaptic receptors in the innervated organ. Phenothiazine antipsychotics such as chlorpromazine and tricyclic antidepressants such as imipramine are derived from antihistamines with a tricyclic structure. It is therefore unsurprising that tricyclic antidepressants act like antihistamines.[1] It is because of this that tricyclic compounds have both antidepressant and sedative effects. Another similarity between antipsychotics and tricyclic antidepressants is the inhibition of acetylcholine receptors,[2] which causes dry mouth, blurred vision, colds and constipation. Another side effect is a drop in blood pressure when standing up suddenly, which is caused by the inhibition of norepinephrine receptors[3] (Gillman 2007; Richelson and Nelson 1984; Whooley and Simon 2000). The effects on dopamine neurotransmission will not be discussed here because they are of limited relevance to the success of antidepressant treatment (Tatsumi et al. 1997).

Because SSRIs have a much more limited effect than tricyclics on neurotransmission through histamine H1 receptors, muscarinic acetylcholine and norepinephrine A1 receptors, their corresponding side effects are also much less severe. Their widespread use in psychiatry and in family and community medicine, however, brought to light a number of important side effects (Cusack et al. 1994; Whooley and Simon 2000; Mann 2005).

The adverse effects of SSRIs are particularly important because their widespread use means they are being prescribed to many patients with mild or moderate depression, or with conditions that, according to the DSM categories already discussed, should not actually be classified as illnesses. The less severe the condition, the less adverse side effects are acceptable. Evidence from their widespread use strongly suggests that SSRIs cause bleeding, sexual dysfunction, discontinuation syndrome and a number of other problems when taken with other medicines, during pregnancy or while breastfeeding.

An examination of the available scientific literature in databases such as PubMed shows a stark contrast between the enormous number of studies and trials on the use of SSRIs and the extremely limited number of studies on their adverse effects. The risk of suicide is by far the most widely discussed and studied area. But it is necessary to examine the evidence of the adverse effects of SSRIs in greater depth.

It is widely known that there is a risk of bleeding in patients treated with SSRIs. In terms of SSRIs' action mechanism, this can be traced to their effect on platelets in the blood. These corpuscles contain many features connected to serotonin, such as monoamine oxidases, many different receptors and the serotonin transporter.

This was the basis for a study on platelets as a model system of neurones in depression (Healy and Leonard 1987). The inhibition of the serotonin transporter disrupts the platelets' involvement in blood coagulation, which causes bleeding. This mainly occurs in the digestive system, and may be more severe in patients with hereditary blood-clotting defects. This also occurs in patients using other medicinal drugs that act on the platelets, such as aspirin and non-steroidal anti-inflammatory agents.

As well as interacting with aspirin and non-steroidal anti-inflammatory agents, SSRIs may also interact with a range of other drugs, essentially because they inhibit hepatic cytochrome. This enzyme is responsible for drug metabolism, and may also significantly modify the efficacy and toxicity of many compounds. The interactions between antidepressants and other drugs should be considered carefully because many people—particularly the elderly—take numerous medicines simultaneously (Serebruany 2006; Weinrieb et al. 2005). The interactions caused by the inhibition of drug metabolism indicate just how carefully they should be considered, and in polytherapy it is essential that prescribers choose the antidepressant that inhibits hepatic cytochrome the least (Hemeryck and Belpaire 2002; DeVane 2006).

SSRIs should be prescribed with caution to women during pregnancy and breastfeeding, in order to limit the exposure of foetuses and newborn babies. Generally, SSRIs are well tolerated and only pose limited risks, but these risks do exist and their impact has not been widely examined, particularly in connection to the neurocognitive development of children. However, there are a number of conditions that often arise during and after pregnancy—in particular, depression—that may require treatment with antidepressants. In these circumstances, treatment has to be carried out with the most scrupulous joint assessment of the risks and benefits for mother and baby (Field 2010; Sie et al. 2012).

Sexual dysfunction is another problem that can arise from the use of SSRIs. The incidence of this side effect is difficult to assess reliably, but the available estimates put it between 30 and 50 %—sometimes even higher. The problem mostly affects men, but many female cases are also reported. The most commonly reported problems are reduced libido, delayed ejaculation and orgasms, and an inability to climax (Ashton Keller et al. 1997; Balon 2006; Fava and Rankin 2002; Kennedy and Rizvi 2009; Prabhakar and Balon 2010).

Another often under-reported problem is what is termed "discontinuation syndrome", which occurs when SSRIs stop being taken. When a treatment of one to two months or more is abruptly interrupted, a significant percentage of patients—estimated by the available literature to be at least 20%—suffer unpleasant physical and psychological effects within a few days. The most common are similar to influenza: insomnia, nausea, lethargy, dizziness, headache, loss of balance, sensory disorders and excitability. These symptoms usually lessen in the following weeks and disappear if treatment is resumed (Haddad 1998; Warner et al. 2006).

The difficulties encountered when taking SSRIs relate back to the problem of psychotropic drug addiction and substance abuse: interrupting the use of these substances quickly leads to abstinence syndrome with serious psychological and physical effects. Benzodiazepine anxiolytics in particular cause withdrawal symptoms, and as a result it is essential that prescribers take care to avoid unjustifiably prolonged use and the abrupt interruption of treatment. The dependence and withdrawal symptoms benzodiazepines cause have often been described as analogous to psychotropic substance abuse. In the case of SSRIs, which are now widely used as an alternative anxiety treatment, the term "discontinuation symptom" is now used much in the same way as "withdrawal" and "dependence" were used for benzodiazepines (WHO 2003). In reality, the effect of discontinuing use is similar for both substances, as confirmed by authoritative sources:

> Withdrawal reactions to selective serotonin re-uptake inhibitors appear to be similar to those for benzodiazepines; referring to these reactions as part of a dependence syndrome in the case of benzodiazepines, but not selective serotonin re-uptake inhibitors, does not seem rational. (Nielsen et al. 2012)

An important matter to consider here is the risk of suicide. This is an extremely severe but relatively uncommon risk arising from the use of SSRIs; it is real risk, however, and is recognised by the FDA, the regulatory body in the USA. There is a large amount of evidence available connecting depression and suicide: in essence, a large number of those who commit suicide suffer from a depressive disorder. The incidence of suicide in those suffering from a depressive disorder is also much higher than in the general population. The question that immediately arises is whether, if a depressed subject receives antidepressant treatment, the suicide risk decreases correspondingly (Ludwig and Marcotte 2005; Hawton et al. 2013). Surprisingly, while it might be expected that antidepressant treatments would reduce the risk of suicide, in the case of SSRIs, there has actually been extensive debate about the question of whether they do not actually *elevate* the suicide risk in patients.

Considering this, it's significant that in 2007 the FDA made it mandatory for all antidepressant packaging to communicate the elevated risk of suicidal tendencies in adults aged between 18 and 24. Since 2004 there has been a similar obligation to warn that the use of antidepressants causes a greater risk of suicidal mood, thoughts and behaviour in children and adolescents. The warning also had to indicate that there is not an increased suicide rate for adults aged between 24 and 65, and that it diminishes for those over 65. The warning, however, contains the assertion that depression and other serious psychiatric disorders are associated with an increased suicide risk, which for the first time explicitly connects the disease and the risk, thus implying that opting out of medicine is also risky.

These warnings became obligatory because of the extensive work of an FDA committee of experts. Their conclusions were published with meta-analysis of data from 372 randomised clinical trials conducted by 12 pharmaceutical companies on almost 100,000 participants. The results suggested the risk increased by 2.2 times in children and adolescents, and by 1.55 times in youths aged 18–24. The risk drops in older age bands and reaches 0.39 times in the over 65 s. The considerable amount of data gave credibility to the meta-analysis, despite several weaknesses. The most important criticism was to do with the data from the short-term clinical trials, which did not take into account long-term safety, obviously of crucial importance (Friedman and Leon 2007).

The analysis suggested that significant numbers of youths are treated in the USA, and this raises the question of how many are really suffering from mental illnesses, and how many are suffering from the passing discomforts typical of childhood and adolescence. The increased suicide risk is even more serious if it is not offset by dependably effective antidepressant treatment. An interesting question would be whether the obligatory FDA warning has changed the use of antidepressants in the USA, and whether this has affected the number of suicidal symptoms. A recent review of the available data suggests that, overall, there has been a decrease in the volume of antidepressants prescribed and the incidence of major depressive disorder since the warning was made obligatory in 2004 (Friedman 2014). However, the relationship between changes in antidepressant use and suicides, suicidal ideation and non-fatal poisoning are complex and the conclusions uncertain (Stone 2014).

There are significant methodological difficulties in conducting studies into whether SSRIs increase suicide risk. Much has been published on this matter, however. The approaches used include meta-analysis, randomised trials and observational and ecological studies: each of these has its strengths and weaknesses, and all provide different evidence. Essentially, the meta-analytical studies suggest that antidepressants cause an increase in suicidal ideation, but this is not specific to SSRIs and is generally limited, meaning there is an acceptable risk-benefit ratio for adults. The risk-benefit ratio for children and adolescents, however, is uncertain in every case except fluoxetine, and in the first few weeks of treatment, close monitoring of suicidal ideation is essential (Hall 2006). In the studies of suicide risk in children and adolescents treated with SSRIs, there is also the problem of unpublished data. When both the published and the unpublished data were examined, the ratio between suicide risk and therapeutic benefit shifted against all antidepressants except fluoxetine. The authors therefore felt it necessary to emphasise the need for greater openness and transparency in all pharmacotherapeutic studies (Whittington et al. 2004).

Notes

1. Inhibition occurring through antagonism with the histamine H1 receptors.
2. Inhibition occurring through antagonism with muscarinic acetylcholine receptors.
3. Orthostatic or supine hypertension occurring via antagonism with norepinephrine A1 receptors.

References

Ashton Keller, A., Hamer, R., & Rosen, R. C. (1997). Serotonin reuptake inhibitor-induced sexual dysfunction and its treatment: A large-scale retrospective study of 596 psychiatric outpatients. *Journal of Sex and Marital Therapy, 23*(3), 165–175.

Balon, R. (2006). SSRI-associated sexual dysfunction. *American Journal of Psychiatry, 163*(9), 1504–1509.

Boyer, E. W., & Shannon, M. (2005). The serotonin syndrome. *New England Journal of Medicine, 352*(11), 1112–1120.

Cusack, B., Nelson, A., & Richelson, E. (1994). Binding of antidepressants to human brain receptors: Focus on newer generation compounds. *Psychopharmacology, 114*(4), 559–565.

DeVane, C. L. (2006). Antidepressant-drug interactions are potentially but rarely clinically significant. *Neuropsychopharmacology, 31*(8), 1594–1604.

Fava, M., & Rankin, M. R. (2002). Sexual functioning and SSRIs. *Journal of Clinical Psychiatry, 63*(5), 13–16.

Field, T. (2010). Prenatal depression and selective serotonin reuptake inhibitors. *International Journal of Neurosciences, 120*(3), 163–167.

Freedman, R. (2003). Schizophrenia. *New England Journal of Medicine, 349*(18), 1738–1749.

Friedman, R. A. (2014). Antidepressants' black-box warning-10 years later. *New England Journal of Medicine, 371*(18), 1666–1668.

Friedman, R. A., & Leon, A. C. (2007). Expanding the black box—depression, antidepressants, and the risk of suicide. *New England Journal of Medicine, 356*(23), 2343–2346.

Gillman, P. K. (2007). Tricyclic antidepressant pharmacology and therapeutic drug interactions updated. *British Journal of Pharmacology, 151*(6), 737–748.

Haddad, P. (1998). The SSRI discontinuation syndrome. *Journal of Psychopharmacology, 12*(3), 305–313.

Hall, W. D. (2006). How have the SSRI antidepressants affected suicide risk? *Lancet, 367*(9527), 1959–1962.

Hawton, K., Casañas, I., Comabella, C., Haw, C., & Saunders, K. (2013). Risk factors for suicide in individuals with depression: A systematic review. *Journal of Affective Disorders, 147*(1–3), 17–28.

Healy, D., & Leonard, B. E. (1987). Monoamine transport in depression: kinetics and dynamics. *Journal of Affective Disorders, 12*(2), 91–103.

Hemeryck, A., & Belpaire, F. M. (2002). Selective serotonin reuptake inhibitors and cytochrome P-450 mediated drug-drug interactions: An update. *Current Drug Metabolism, 3*(1), 13–37.

Kennedy, S. H., & Rizvi, S. (2009). Sexual dysfunction, depression, and the impact of antidepressants. *Journal of Clinical Psychopharmacology, 29*(2), 157–164.

Ludwig, J., & Marcotte, D. E. (2005). Anti-depressants, suicide, and drug regulation. *Journal of Policy Analysis and Management, 24*(2), 249–272.

Mann, J. J. (2005). The medical management of depression. *New England Journal of Medicine, 353*(17), 1819–1834.

Meyer, U. A. (2000). Pharmacogenetics and adverse drug reactions. *Lancet, 356*(9242), 1667–1671.

Nielsen, M., Hansen, E. H., & Gøtzsche, P. C. (2012). What is the difference between dependence and withdrawal reactions? A comparison of benzodiazepines and selective serotonin re-uptake inhibitors. *Addiction, 107*(5), 900–908.

Prabhakar, D., & Balon, R. (2010). How do SSRIs cause sexual dysfunction. *Current Psychiatry, 9*(12), 30–35.

Richelson, E., & Nelson, A. (1984). Antagonism by antidepressants of neurotransmitter receptors of normal human brain in vitro. *Journal of Pharmacology and Experimental Therapeutics, 230*(1), 94–102.

Serebruany, V. L. (2006). Selective serotonin reuptake inhibitors and increased bleeding risk: Are we missing something? *American Journal of Medicine, 119*(2), 113–116.

Shulman, K. I., Herrmann, N., & Walker, S. E. (2013). Current place of monoamine oxidase inhibitors in the treatment of depression. *CNS Drugs, 27*(10), 789–797.

Sie, S. D., Wennink, J. M., van Driel, J. J., te Winkel, A.G., Boer, K., Casteelen, G., & van Weissenbruch, M. M. (2012). Maternal use of SSRIs, SNRIs and NaSSAs: Practical recommendations during pregnancy and lactation. *Archives of Disease in Childhood. Fetal and Neonatal Edition, 97*(6), F472–F476.

Stone, M. B. (2014). The FDA warning on antidepressants and suicidality-why the controversy? *New England Journal of Medicine, 371*(18), 1668–1671.

Tatsumi, M., Groshan, K., Blakely, R. D., & Richelson, E. (1997). Pharmacological profile of antidepressants and related compounds at human monoamine transporters. *European Journal of Pharmacology, 340*(2–3), 249–258.

Warner, C. H., Bobo, W., Warner, C., Reid, S., & Rachal, J. (2006). Antidepressant discontinuation syndrome. *American Family Physician, 74*(3), 449–456.

Weinrieb, R. M., Auriacombe, M., Lynch, K. G., & Lewis, J. D. (2005). Selective serotonin re-uptake inhibitors and the risk of bleeding. *Expert Opinion in Drug Safety, 4*(2), 337–344.

Whittington, C. J., Kendall, T., Fonagy, P., Cottrell, D., Cotgrove, A., & Boddington. E. (2004). Selective serotonin reuptake inhibitors in childhood depression: Systematic review of published versus unpublished data. *Lancet, 363*(9418), 1341–1345.

WHO. (2003). WHO Expert Committee on Drug Dependence: Thirty-third Report (Vol. 33). http://apps.who.int/iris/bitstream/10665/42655/1/WHO_TRS_915.pdf. Accessed 30 May, 2016.

Whooley, M. A., & Simon, G. E. (2000). Managing depression in medical outpatients. *New England Journal of Medicine, 343*(26), 1942–1950.

12

Conclusion

Our great struggle in medicine these days is not just with ignorance and uncertainty. It's also with complexity: how much you have to make sure you have in your head and think about. There are a thousand ways things can go wrong.
Atul Gawande

In the years after the end of the Second World War, extraordinary advances were made in our understanding of the electrochemical phenomena responsible for brain function. A vital part of this was coming to understand the transmission of nerve impulses between neurones, nerves and muscles. The neurotransmitters involved were identified, along with the processes through which they are synthesised in the nerve cells and released in response to nerve impulses. We also came to understand how they act on innervated cells by triggering a response to the nerve impulse, later leading back to the initial state of rest. Advances in our understanding of these mechanisms were coupled with the birth of psychopharmacology, which came about because of the identification of families of compounds that act on the brain, and this also contributed to our understanding of the brain's functions. Psychopharmacology has changed the face of mental institutions and psychiatry, which until

© The Author(s) 2017
T. Giraldi, *Unhappiness, Sadness and 'Depression'*,
DOI 10.1007/978-3-319-57657-2_12

then had neither a sound understanding of the mechanisms behind mental illness nor effective drugs to treat it. The birth of psychopharmacology also had a social impact outside the world of psychiatry.

The first drugs involved in this revolution were meprobamate and benzodiazepines, which were then called minor tranquilisers. Paradoxically, however, they actually had the greatest impact *outside* psychiatry. The risk of acute poisoning, which had been a serious problem with barbiturates such as sedatives and hypnotics, was negligible with benzodiazepines, and because of this and their pleasant effects, they soon came to be used in general medicine—and through self-prescription—to help people relieve the stress of everyday life. Benzodiazepines were soon in widespread use, but this decreased significantly when their patent expired and more emphasis was placed on their tendency to induce tolerance and dependence.

The antipsychotic drugs used to treat schizophrenia, on the other hand, were to have a radical effect on psychiatric practice and even the organisation and appearance of mental institutions. Because of their pronounced side effects, however, these drugs are now used only for more severe cases of mental suffering. A similar thing also happened to the drugs used to treat manic depression, now called bipolar disorder.

This did not happen, however, in the case of antidepressants. The remarkable effects of the first tricyclic derivatives and monoamine oxidase inhibitors were obvious right from the start. The therapeutic effects on depression sufferers were irrefutable. From the perspective of pharmaceutical companies, however, the number of people suffering from what was formerly known as endogenous or vital depression was so small that the market did not seem profitable enough to justify research into new derivatives. This changed dramatically, however, when selective serotonin reuptake inhibitors (SSRIs) became available. They were prescribed so widely that they joined the very select group of medicines that have generated outstanding revenues both during and after their patent validity. It's important to consider how this came about.

The first factor behind the increase in the number of people treated with SSRIs is that these drugs have much less severe side effects. The chemical structure of tricyclic antidepressants is very similar to first generation phenothiazine antipsychotics, and as a result they share a number of severe and sometimes irreversible side effects—fortunately not including motor disorders. The pronounced side effects of tricyclic antidepressants were only acceptable when treating severe cases of depression, because the benefits outweighed the risks. Fluoxetine and its SSRI analogues, however, were another matter altogether. Their new chemical structure and action mechanism caused decidedly less common and pronounced side effects. The increased tolerability of SSRIs and their improved risk-benefit ratio meant they could be used for milder forms of mood disorder, as well as other conditions such as obsessive compulsive disorder, panic attacks and eating disorders.

They could also be prescribed much more widely, although unlike benzodiazepine anxiolytics, there was no self-prescription trend. It was not just psychiatrists who prescribed SSRIs, however: many family doctors also started to prescribe them. This was possible, essentially, because the diagnostic criteria were extended to include mild and moderate depression, and this corresponded with changes to the diagnostic criteria in the *Diagnostic and Statistical Manual of Mental Disorders* (DSM). The arrival of the DSM-5 drew serious criticism from Thomas Insel, the Director of the National Institute of Mental Health (NIMH) in the USA. He criticised its limitations on his blog on the NIMH website: 'Patients with mental disorders deserve better'. Insel added that the DSM's diagnostic categories are based on a cluster of symptoms, and that:

> In the rest of medicine, this would be equivalent to creating diagnostic systems based on the nature of chest pain or the quality of fever. Indeed, symptom-based diagnosis, once common in other areas of medicine, has been largely replaced in the past half century as we have understood that symptoms alone rarely indicate the best choice of treatment.

NIMH soon launched the Research Domain Criteria (RDoC) project to transform psychiatric diagnosis, research and treatment and create a new classification system incorporating genetics, cognitive sciences and modern brain-imaging techniques (Insel 2013).

The nature and extension of the diagnostic criteria for depression have led to the perception that depression includes both major depressive disorders and ever-milder forms of mood disorder, which are often non-pathological in nature or even "normal" emotions or mood states. Because the diagnostic criteria were extended, ever-greater volumes of antidepressants were soon being prescribed.

More SSRI antidepressants are being prescribed partly because of pressure from the pharmaceutical industry, and partly because of the procedures for authorising the marketing of new antidepressants. New drugs can now be authorised by providing results from a limited number of clinical trials sponsored and effectively conducted by pharmaceutical companies. Pharmaceutical companies do not even have to publish all their results: they can keep them secret and simply choose the studies they want published. In fact, all studies need to show is that a new compound causes a modest reduction on the psychometric scale compared to placebos. It is not necessary to show they are more or even equally as effective as the drugs already on the market. New drugs are therefore authorised for market on the basis of only modest clinical efficacy. This may pose problems for prescribers when dealing with severe depression, because many new drugs are authorised without being tested on more serious cases. Understandably, therefore, many prescribers still resort to tricyclic antidepressants for more severe depression, because there is extensive evidence of their effectiveness in these cases.

There has been remarkable pressure from drug manufacturers to extend the use of antidepressants, which even shows in today's diagnostic criteria. These determine not only how diseases are categorised but also how drugs are prescribed and whether the costs of antidepressants and other medicines can be reimbursed. In 2006, Lisa Cosgrove analysed the remarkable conflicts of interest arising because DSM-IV panel members had financial connections with industry sponsors (Cosgrove et al. 2006). In further analysis carried out in 2012 she observed that:

> The APA instituted a financial conflict of interest disclosure policy for the 5th edition of the DSM, the new policy has not been accompanied by a reduction in the financial conflicts of interest of DSM panel members. Transparency alone cannot mitigate the potential for bias and is an insufficient solution for protecting the integrity of the revision process. Gaps in the disclosure policy are identified and recommendations for more stringent safeguards are offered. (Cosgrove and Krimsky 2012)

The pressure from the pharmaceutical industry to increase the size of the antidepressant market is substantial, and has been the subject of repeated and thorough analysis. The in-depth analysis in Marcia Angell's 2004 book has already been mentioned, but there are many other investigations into how the pressure to prescribe medicines has gradually eroded cornerstone principles such as ethical and scientific values. These principles have gradually been replaced by modern marketing techniques and the economic strength of the pharmaceutical industry.

Depression is a perfect example of how diagnostic criteria have been expanded to include more and more subtle and less detectable symptoms. In parallel with this, treatments have become objectively less safe and effective. There is an extensive amount of literature available on this, and it will be useful to refer to some of the best scientific publications on the matter. Lynn Payer used the term "disease-mongers" in her book *Disease-Mongers: How Doctors, Drug Companies, and Insurers are Making You Feel Sick* (Payer 1992). In his book *Selling Sickness: How the World's Biggest Pharmaceutical Companies are Turning Us all into Patients* (Moynihan and Cassels 2005), Ray Moynihan is equally interested in the idea of new diseases being created in order to prescribe medicines. In particular, Moynihan analyses how minor and temporary issues in women's sex lives can be turned into morbid conditions. He describes how a new syndrome—female sexual dysfunction—came to be included in the DSM (Moynihan 2003), and how a wide array of drugs were rapidly developed to treat it (Moynihan 2005). The problem of female sexual dysfunction is an exemplary case, which Moynihan analyses further in his book *Sex, Lies and Pharmaceuticals: How Drug Companies Plan to Profit from Female Sexual Dysfunction* (Moynihan and Mintzes 2010). Jacky Law came to similar conclusions in her book *Big Pharma: How the World's Biggest Drug Companies Control Illness* (Law 2006), as did Jörg Blech in *Inventing Disease and Pushing Pills* (Blech 2006). Andrea Tone's *Medicating Modern America: Prescription Drugs in History* collects a range of contributions examining the concept of disease and its treatment in the modern era, particularly in relation to depression (Tone 2009). Jerome Kassirer also analyses the crucial role played by the medical establishment in his essential work *On the Take: How Medicine's Complicity with Big Business can Endanger Your Health* (Kassirer 2005).

In light of all this, it appears that ethical safeguards and the rigour and validity of scientific data have gradually been eroded. Clinical trials are central to the authorisation of new drugs, but a lack of public access and the impossibility of independent critical assessment mean their organisers are increasingly able to evade scientific scrutiny. In the context of globalisation, multicentric trials are often partially conducted in countries with limited standard care and low levels of protection for the subjects involved. Clinical trials that were previously conducted in university clinics or highly specialised, renowned hospitals in developed countries are increasingly outsourced and carried out by private, profit-driven companies that pay their subjects to take part. This new arrangement is increasingly problematic, often lowering the standard and rigour of the scientists performing the trials and the volunteers selected.

There are other worrying new developments too, such as the formation of independent ethics committees and institutional review boards (IRBs), which have a crucial role in authorising clinical trials. They play a vital part because they should only allow the authorisation of new drugs when pre-clinical studies suggest the safety and efficacy of the drugs will justify the risks for volunteers. They should also only authorise trials that will lead to significant therapeutic progress, based on valid experimental protocols. When pre-clinical studies are conducted at higher-education institutes, the ethics committees of those same institutes generally decide whether to authorise further trials. These committees are usually rigorous and ethical. US regulations currently require pre-clinical studies to be reviewed by one ethics committee, which does not have to be from the institution where the trials will take place. Because it is possible to effectively outsource authorisation, numerous companies have been formed with the sole purpose of carrying out reviews to authorise clinical trials. This leaves room for deficient and possibly fraudulent behaviour, as the US Government Accountability Office (GAO) confirmed in 2009. The GAO conducted an investigation in which they were able to gain state accreditation for a non-existent IRB. By submitting fictitious documentation to a real commercial IRB, they were also able to get permission to begin clinical trials for a fake product, Adhesiabloc (GAO 2009; Elliott 2010).

There have been studies on the same authority and integrity of mechanisms of scientific communication, and publication of results in scientific journals, which indicated the emergence of undesirable situations over time, which compromise the neutrality and fairness of the peer review system[1] and require suitable corrections. Richard Smith, the long-time editor of the authoritative *British Medical Journal*, has outlined on the basis of his own experiences aspects of the publishing process in medical journals which require attention and correction. Among the major problems, Smith cites conflicts of interest and relations between medical journals, the mass media and pharmaceutical companies, calling them "moving from love and hate to love", and "uneasy bedfellows" (Smith 2006).

The presence of honorary and ghost authors numbers among the problems related to scientific publications, since they confer importance to the articles published through their authority, without having participated in the study to any extent. The scale of the phenomenon is widespread, estimated at 39% for honorary authors and 11% for ghost authors, in a large sample of medical journals. In 2008, of the six journals of greatest medical impact, 21% of the articles published comprised honorary or ghost authors, indicating the need to take corrective measures (Wislar et al. 2011). There are aspects of the publishing process of biomedical journals which require adequate correction measures, as would appear from the position taken by the recent winner of the Nobel Prize for Medicine and Physiology, Randy Schekman. He publicly stated that he will boycott publications in the best-known biology and medicine journals such as *Nature*, *Cell* and *Science*. Schekman has complained of a sort of tyranny exercised by these journals, who create distortions in the functioning of the world of research and scientific communication; the editors of the journals concerned have voiced their reactions (*The Guardian* 2013).

There has been much criticism of the current clinical research processes for authorising new medicines, some of which has already been mentioned. Ben Goldacre has repeatedly highlighted the scientific limitations of these processes, pointing to examples of the deficient design of clinical trials, the inaccessibility and possible manipulation of their results, and the growing role of marketing (Goldacre 2012). A particular example of this was a campaign in Japan in the early 2000s. It was sponsored by the manufacturer of the SSRI antidepressant paroxetine, which had previously made scarcely any sales in the country. Because of this intensive campaign, much of the stigma attached to depression[2] in Japan has dissipated, and it is now often referred to in Japanese as a "cold of the soul".[3] As a result, the manufacturer has since seen a marked increase in sales (Watters 2010).

The model that enabled the extraordinary growth of the North American and European pharmaceutical industries after the Second World War seems today to be in crisis. The great success of the pharmaceutical industry was based on the identification of innovative molecular entities which changed the world of medicine and generated immense profits. The most profitable—like antidepressants—were termed "blockbusters". Despite the efforts of multinational drug companies, as well as major advances in basic sciences, biomedicine and neuroscience, however, the number of new compounds being authorised for market is currently stagnant. This is particularly true for drugs that affect the nervous system, to the extent that pharmaceutical companies are abandoning this once highly profitable sector.

Thomas Insel has proposed a number of possible solutions to this. First, under his directorship it's expected that NIMH will adopt new approaches to organising and financing their research. New clinical trials will need to adopt an experimental medical approach aimed at identifying new possible treatments. They will also need to produce information on the mechanisms behind disorders, identify new drug targets and take into account the psychosocial aspects of disorders. Future trials will need to meet new standards of efficacy and transparency to overcome delays, limited public access and bias in publications. One of the motivations for these changes is the realisation that the process of identifying new drugs has withered after decades of producing "me-too" drugs (Insel 2014; Reardon 2014; Editorial Nature 2014). NIMH's new approach also anticipates a shift away from using animal experimentation for psychiatric drugs, and towards the translation of basic studies into clinical research. This research would include trials based on realistic assessment criteria which take into account the real lives of patients. No risk factors have yet been identified in genetic-molecular research, and this could also help to promote the identification of the biological indicators of disease, as well as new targets for innovative drug developments.

The fact that NIMH's new research approach will take into account the psychosocial dimensions of disorders seems particularly interesting. It recalls the fact that, in the absence of drugs, depression and anxiety—which were previously understood as "neurotic" conditions—were first treated psychologically with the "talking cure". The methods of medical treatment are normally indicated in guidelines drafted at national, continental or international levels by professional associations of medical specialists. In the case of treatments for depression, antidepressants became more common and accepted because of the influence of the USA and the American Psychiatric Association (APA). The authoritative advisory body in the UK is the National Institute for Health and Clinical Excellence (NICE), which is geared at producing accurate guidelines on the main therapeutic approaches. NICE has repeatedly considered all the evidence available on antidepressants and released detailed guidelines for their use. It's significant that the NICE guidelines explicitly state that antidepressants should not be used routinely for cases of mild or moderate depression if there is a low risk-benefit ratio. In these cases, it suggests a stepped-care intervention model, which can be intensified depending on the severity of the condition and guided by the patient's preference for:

- Self-help guided by the principles of cognitive behavioural therapy
- Cognitive behavioural therapy
- Group physical activity within a structured programme.

Antidepressants should be proposed if these treatments are ineffective, if mild symptoms have persisted for years or if the patient has already suffered episodes of severe depression. In the case of moderate to severe depression, a combination of antidepressant pharmacotherapy and "high-intensity" psychological intervention is recommended

(NICE 2009). The matter of intervention for children and adolescents is considered separately, and a gradual stepped-care approach is recommended. It also suggests the limited use of drugs for severe cases, after careful consideration of the family environment and the relationships around the patient (NICE 2009).

The UK's National Health Service (NHS) adopted these guidelines and also initially invested £400 million into the Improving Access to Psychological Therapy (IAPT) programme. Launched in 2011, this 4-year programme was designed to bring the NHS's training and structures into line with NICE's depression treatment guidelinesy (Talking Therapies 2011; IAPT 2015a). The results in the first 3 years were extremely positive. Over a million people underwent treatment and 680,000 completed it. Over 45% of the subjects completely recovered, 65% improved significantly and the improvements observed were more stable than those before: overall, more than 45,000 people returned to work. 4000 new staff members were trained, and the NHS's mental health services are being widely restructured. Other European countries are adopting similar methods and observing similarly positive results (IAPT 2012).

The results of the IAPT are significant because they involve large numbers of people participating in a national-scale project. Numerous studies carried out on smaller groups of patients also suggest that cognitive behavioural psychotherapy and psychosocial support—either on their own or combined with other treatments—are effective for mood disorders of varying severity, and that the resulting improvements are generally more stable (Linde et al. 2015a).

It's worth noting here that in the world of medicine, psychotherapy has become almost synonymous with cognitive behavioural therapy (CBT). This treatment was developed by Aaron Beck (Beck 1987), who first showed its effectiveness (Whitfield and Williams 2003). It was one of the many psychotherapeutic approaches developed in the wake of Sigmund Freud. But is CBT the only form of psychotherapy effective against depression, or are there others? Meta-analysis was carried out into this very question. It considered the effectiveness of CBT, psychodynamic psychotherapy based on psychoanalytics, other more general forms of psychotherapy, and pharmacotherapy with antidepressants.

The results suggested that all the psychotherapies were actually equally effective. They also showed that antidepressants were only about half as effective as psychotherapy in most cases (Shedler 2010).

More extended meta-analysis was conducted on the effects of psychotherapy and pharmacotherapy on a range of psychiatric disorders. The results were mostly inconclusive, but they showed that psychotherapy and combined treatment were generally more effective than pharmacotherapy alone in the case of depression (Huhn et al. 2014). When the results of particularly rigorous studies—which included complementary alternative medicine (CAM) as well as pharmacotherapy and psychotherapy—were considered, it was found that a combination of drugs and psychotherapy was most effective. It was also found that the individual treatments considered did not have significantly different effects to the group treatments. Outside depression, the evidence suggests the modest but significant efficacy of pharmacotherapy (Linde et al. 2015b) compared to psychological interventions, which seem to be less effective (Linde et al. 2015b).

It seems that mild and moderate depression can be treated successfully with other methods besides antidepressants. As well as psychotherapy, studies have found a number of other approaches can also be effective. Mindfulness is a particularly interesting example, both because of its conceptual foundations and because of the evidence for its effectiveness. Jon Kabat-Zinn first proposed meditation as a way of alleviating the symptoms of anxiety and depression. Originally a biologist, Kabat-Zinn shifted his attention to meditation and, in 1979, he founded the Stress Reduction Clinic, later the Center for Mindfulness in Medicine, Health Care, and Society, at the Medical School of Massachusetts University. Kabat-Zinn's interest soon developed into a real programme called Mindfulness-Based Stress Reduction (MBSR), which soon became widespread in the USA and other countries (Kabat-Zinn 1991).

One of Kabat-Zinn's most recent books concerns depression in particular, and its purpose is clearly indicated in the title: *The Mindful Way Through Depression: Freeing Yourself from Chronic Unhappiness* (Williams et al. 2007). Kabat-Zinn's approach is certainly not aimed at those affected by severe mental illnesses. It recalls the relationship between stress and depression, or rather how the difficulty of adapting to stressful life events may translate into emotions and disturbed moods. The idea of identifying ways to tackle and reduce the negative effects of stress is not new: one example is Herbert Benson's (1975) proposal for a programme called "The Relaxation Response". It aimed to alleviate stress and anxiety through transcendental meditation, which had been developed by Maharishi Mahesh Yogi (Benson 1975) and was in vogue at the time. Kabat-Zinn's work, on the other hand, was based on the age-old practice of Buddhist meditation, which is based on rigorous methods that have been analysed in a number of scientific works (Brewer et al. 2011).

Like Aaron Beck with cognitive behavioural psychotherapy, Kabat-Zinn was committed to showing the effectiveness of mindfulness with something more than anecdotal evidence (Hofmann et al. 2010; Brewer et al. 2011). Of course, unhappiness and sadness are outside the realms of evidence-based medicine, but Kabat-Zinn's meditation programme has nevertheless been shown to be effective in the treatment of psoriasis (Kabat-Zinn et al. 1998) and tobacco addiction in chronic smokers. In the latter, the effects of mindfulness are specific and independent of the relaxation induced by meditation (Tang et al. 2013).

From these studies, it seems there is an opportunity to differentiate between cases of serious mental suffering, which require intensive intervention—sometimes involving antidepressants—and non-morbid states of unhappiness and distress resulting from challenging life situations. In severe depression, therefore, antidepressants may be an effective tool for overcoming serious episodes. Psychological support and psychotherapy may also add to these results. The improvements caused by this approach are also generally more stable over time because they rely on generating a better response to life events and to the emotions that may accompany them. Mindfulness meditation—with its efficacy and lack of adverse effects—is increasingly seen as a useful tool to calm the mind. It is no longer viewed as just a New Age alternative but rather a serious method with an important part to play in society through schools, the health system and many other areas (Bunting 2014).

A large number of publications about depression and the use of antidepressants continue to appear in scientific journals, and depression continues to be diagnosed—almost invariably—using the DSM's "major depressive disorder" criteria. In every country where studies have been conducted, depression as defined by these criteria is remarkably common in all strata of society, including the old, the young and people of both sexes. In the USA, analysis carried out by the National Center for Health Statistics suggests that antidepressants were the third most common prescription drug taken by Americans of all ages in 2005–2008. They were also the drug most frequently used by persons aged 18–44 years. Between 1988–1994 and 2005–2008 there was almost a 400% increase in the use of antidepressants by people of all ages in the USA. About one in ten Americans aged 12 and over currently takes antidepressant medication. Overall, females are 2.5 times as likely to take antidepressant medication as males, and 23% of women aged 40–59 were found to be on antidepressants—more than any other age-sex group. In both males and females, those aged 40 and over were more likely to take antidepressants than those in younger age groups. While the majority of antidepressants are taken to treat depression, they are also used to treat other disorders such as anxiety (Pratt et al. 2011). In the UK, analysis by the Quality Watch of the Health Foundation of the Nuffield Trust found a 165% increase in the prescription of antidepressants by GPs in England between 1998 and 2012 (Spence et al. 2014). In Italy, the national regulatory agency Agenzia Italiana del Farmaco's (AIFA) annual report of medicine use in 2015 suggested 12.6% of the general population had been diagnosed with depression: 16.8% of women and 9% of men. Antidepressants, mainly SSRIs (21%), were prescribed to 29% of depression sufferers, with a compliance rate of 31.6% (AIFA 2016).

It's also useful to consider the results of a study into antidepressant use in children and adolescents between 2005 and 2012. After the introduction of the Food and Drug Administration's (FDA) black box warning about the risk of suicidal ideation in children and adolescents, there was an initial reduction in use. However, databases from Denmark, Germany, the Netherlands, the UK and the USA show that this did not persist. In fact, in recent years the use of antidepressants by children and adolescents has increased substantially in these countries (Bachmanna et al. 2016). There are still many unanswered questions about diagnosing and treating depression in children using the regulatory procedures developed for adults.

The prevalence of depression and antidepressant medication is high and constantly rising. Antidepressants are in fact much more common than drugs used for the treatment of other serious psychiatric conditions (Ilyas and Moncrieff 2012; Stephenson et al. 2013). Nevertheless, a recent initiative by the US Preventive Services Task Force proposes screening every adult in the USA for depression, and the January 2016 issue of the *Journal of the American Medical Association* published two editorials and two articles supporting the proposal. Surprisingly, one of the articles was even addressed to patients, despite the fact the journal is circulated to doctors. The proposal is accompanied by the suggestion that there should be follow-ups and drug treatments when the screening identifies depression in patients. The diagnostic criteria proposed are even more inclusive than those of the DSM and are essentially based on the use of common psychometric scales such as the Patient Health Questionnaire, the Hospital Anxiety and Depression Scales, the Geriatric Depression Scale and the Edinburgh Postnatal Depression Scale (JAMA 2016).

Allen Frances, the psychiatrist who chaired the task force that prepared the revised edition of the DSM-IV, later criticised its widespread and inappropriate use, and set out his revised position in the book *Saving Normal: An Insider's Revolt against Out-of-Control Psychiatric Diagnosis, DSM-5, Big Pharma, and the Medicalization of Ordinary Life* (Frances 2013). Interviewed by the *New Scientist* about the US Preventive Services Task Force initiative, he called the screening "[a] good intention, a very bad idea" which will "create an army of pseudo-patients while the really sick are shamefully neglected". He expressed his concern about the combination of loose diagnostic criteria in the DSM and aggressive marketing by drug companies, which led to more than 10% of Americans now being on antidepressants, rising to 25% for women over 40, and amounting to an increase of 400% in the past 20 years (Frances 2016).

Concern about the epidemic of depression and inappropriate antidepressant use is not limited to scientific and medical journals. Recently, articles have appeared in the *Guardian* in the UK (The Guardian 2014,

2016), and in the USA posts have been published about the subject on the Harvard Health Blog (Harvard Health Blog 2011). Another noteworthy example is the *New York Review of Books*, which published an issue devoted to the epidemic of mental diseases and its causes, with authoritative editorship by Marcia Angell and reference to the work of Irving Kirsch, Robert Whitaker and Daniel Carlat (The New York Review of Books 2011a, b).

Supporters of the current diagnostic criteria and methods for treating depression continue to publish articles on their views. Kramer added to his list of published works on the subject with *Ordinarily Well: The Case for Antidepressants*. In this book, he once more uses a selection of the available literature to support the most extended use of antidepressants (Kramer 2016). A strongly contrasting position is expressed by Gøtzsche, based on careful and rigorous meta-analysis of all the scientific literature available, made through the Nordic Cochrane Center and the Cochrane Collaboration. He has also publicised his position with recent books on the excess development and extensive use of psychiatric drugs and particularly antidepressants (Gøtzsche et al. 2013; Gøtzsche 2015). Another recent book which is receiving increasing public attention is *The Pill That Steals Lives* by Katinka Blackford Newman, which reports the very serious side effects she suffered during treatment with antidepressant drugs. Blackford Newman, a professional documentary filmmaker, includes interviews with leading UK experts who outline how antidepressant drugs may cause very serious adverse reactions, which are largely underestimated and may substantially harm patients (Blackford Newman 2016).

The IAPT programme is still being implemented, however, and its results continue to be examined. Analysis in 2015 confirmed the positive results that had previously been reported. Several methods of intervention were used. In descending order of recovery rates, they were: computerised cognitive behavioural therapy (CCBT), interpersonal psychotherapy (IPT), couple therapy, guided self-help, brief psychodynamic psychotherapy, counselling, behavioural activation, CBT, psychoeducational peer support and pure self-help. The recovery rates ranged from 58.4 to 38.5% (pure self-help) (IAPT 2015b). The evidence available so far does not suggest significant differences in effectiveness between the seven psychotherapies for adult depression (Barth et al. 2013) and between cognitive and dynamic psychotherapy (Connolly Gibbons et al. 2016). Similarly, in a community mental health setting, behavioural activation was found to be both similarly effective and economical compared to the more complex and costly CBT (Richards et al. 2016). The data available did not show significant differences between "third-wave" cognitive and behavioural therapies and other psychological therapies for depression in adults in a Cochrane review (Hunot et al. 2013). This lack of difference, however, might be attributed to a lack of statistical power in the available studies (Cuijpers 2016). This suggests that it may be necessary to encourage research into the most appropriate treatments for all mood disorders, which might range from support and self-help, to psychotherapy and drug therapy, depending on the characteristics of the disorder to be treated.

All this suggests that it is important for patients to be directly involved in their treatments. A recent study conducted in the Netherlands found that depressed subjects considered the following strategies effective and positive for their conditions:

- Be aware that "my depression" requires "my active intervention" even in the case of professional treatment
- Have an active lifestyle with structured and programmed free time
- Participate daily in social and working life.

During the study—even in relation to CCBT—patients seemed to emphasise the need for face-to-face treatment with their therapist, and for building a long-term relationship with them. They also stressed the need to be sufficiently involved in social and work life and with their family, friends, colleagues and even clinicians (van Grieken et al. 2014).

It is therefore desirable that balanced, humane, serene, effective and safe approaches to the treatment of mood disorders develop and become established. They should be set within a realistic and empathetic framework, and they should avoid reductionist perspectives based on progressive but fragmented knowledge that lacks clinical confirmation. Crucially, as far as possible, they should limit bias from profit-driven lobbyists.

Notes

1. System of evaluation by external experts to determine the value and fairness of research projects or communications and scientific publications.
2. *Ustubyo*, incurable depression.
3. *Kokoro no kaze.*

References

AIFA. (2016). Rapporto sull'uso dei farmaci in Italia. Rapporto nazionale 2015. http://www.agenziafarmaco.gov.it/sites/default/files/Rapporto_OsMed_2015__AIFA.pdf. Accessed 4 Jan 2017.

Bachmanna, C. J., Aagaard, L., Burcu, M., et al. (2016). Trends and patterns of antidepressant use in children and adolescents from five western countries, 2005–2012. *European Neuropsychopharmacology, 26,* 411–419.

Barth, J., Munder, T., Gerger, H., et al. (2013). Comparative efficacy of seven psychotherapeutic interventions for patients with depression: A network meta-analysis. *PLoS Medicine, 10*(5), e1001454. doi:10.1371/journal.pmed.1001454.

Beck, A. T., Rush, A. J., Shaw, B. F., & Emery, G. (1987). *Cognitive therapy of depression.* New York: Guilford Press.

Benson, H. (1975). *The relaxation response.* New York: Avon Books.

Blackford Newman, K. (2016). *The pill that steals lives.* London: John Blake.

Blech, J. (2006). *Inventing disease and pushing dills.* London: Routledge.

Brewer, J. A., Mallik, S., Babuscio, T. A., et al. (2011). Mindfulness training for smoking cessation: Results from a randomized controlled trial. *Drug Alcohol Dependence, 119*(1–2), 72–80.

Bunting, M. (2014). *Why we will come to see mindfulness as mandatory.* http://www.theguardian.com/commentisfree/2014/may/06/mindfulness-hospitals-schools. Accessed 16 Apr 2015.

Connolly Gibbons, M. B., Gallop, R., Thompson, D., et al. (2016). Comparative effectiveness of cognitive therapy and dynamic psychotherapy for major depressive disorder in a community mental health setting: A randomized clinical noninferiority trial. *Journal of the American Medical Association Psychiatry, 73*(9), 904–911.

Cosgrove, L., & Krimsky, S. (2012). A comparison of DSM-IV and DSM-5 panel members' financial associations with industry: A pernicious

problem persists. *PLoS Medicine, 9*(3), e1001190. doi:10.1371/journal.
pmed.1001190.

Cosgrove, L., Krimsky, S., Vijayaraghavan, M., et al. (2006). Financial
ties between DSM-IV panel members and the pharmaceutical industry.
Psychotherapy and Psychosomatics, 75(3), 154–160.

Cuijpers, P. (2016). Are all psychotherapies equally effective in the treatment of
adult depression? The lack of statistical power of comparative outcome studies. *Evidence-Based Mental Health, 19*(2), 39–42.

Editorial Nature. (2014). What lies beneath. A focus on specific biological
targets rather than constellations of symptoms heralds a more scientific
approach to the treatment of neuropsychiatric disorders. *Nature, 507*(273).
doi:10.1038/507273a.

Elliott, C. (2010). *White Coat, Black Hat.* Boston: Beacon Press.

Frances, A. (2013) Saving Normal: An Insider's Revolt Against Out-Of-
Control Psychiatric Diagnosis, Dsm-5, Big Pharma, and the Medicalization
of Ordinary Life. New York: William Morrow, an imprint of HarperCollins
publishers.

Frances, A. (2016, January 26). Screen everyone for depression? Good intention, very bad idea. New Scientist. Comment. https://www.newscientist.
com/article/2075249-screen-everyone-for-depression-good-intention-very-
bad-idea/. Accessed 4 Jan 2017.

GAO. U.S. Government Accountability Office. (2009). *Human subjects
research: Undercover tests show the Institutional Review Board system is vulnerable to unethical manipulation.* http://www.gao.gov/new.items/d09448t.pdf.
Accessed 11 Apr 2015.

Goetzsche, P. (2015). *Deadly psychiatry and organized denial.* København:
People's Press.

Goldacre, B. (2012). *Bad medicine. How drug companies mislead doctors and
harm patients.* London, Fourth Estate.

Gøtzsche, P. C., Smith, R., & Drummond, R. (2013). *Deadly medicines and
organised crime: How big pharma has corrupted healthcare.* London: Radcliffe
Publishing.

Harvard Health Blog. (2011, October 20). *Astounding increase in antidepressant
use by Americans.* Peter Wehrwein. Retrieved January 4, 2017, from http://
www.health.harvard.edu/blog/astounding-increase-in-antidepressant-use-
by-americans-201110203624.

Hofmann, S. G., Sawyer, A. T., Witt, A. A., & Oh, D. (2010). The effect of
mindfulness-based therapy on anxiety and depression: A meta-analytic
review. *Journal of Consulting and Clinical Psychology, 78*(2), 69–83.

12 Conclusion 183

Huhn, M., Tardy, M., Spineli, L. M., et al. (2014). Efficacy of pharmaco-therapy and psychotherapy for adult psychiatric disorders: A systematic overview of meta-analyses. *The Journal of American Medical Association. Psychiatry, 71*(6), 706–715.

Hunot, V., Moore, T. H., Caldwell, D. M. et al. (2013). *'Third wave' cognitive and behavioural therapies versus other psychological therapies for depression.* Cochrane Database of Systematic Reviews 2013, Issue 10. Art. No.: CD008704. doi:10.1002/14651858.CD008704.pub2. http://onlinelibrary.wiley.com/doi/10.1002/14651858.CD008704.pub2/abstract;jsessionid=4C0109A49619D5B64123E345B73AE12F.f03t03. Accessed 4, 4 Jan 2017.

IAPT. (2012). *Supporting no health without mental health.* https://www.gov.uk/government/uploads/system/uploads/attachment_data/file/216870/No-Health-Without-Mental-Health-Implementation-Framework-Report-accessible-version.pdf. Accessed 15 Apr 2015.

IAPT. (2015a). *Improving access to psychological therapies.* https://www.england.nhs.uk/mentalhealth/adults/iapt/. Accessed 4 Jan 2017.

IAPT. (2015b). *Psychological therapies; annual report on the use of IAPT services: England 2014/15.* http://content.digital.nhs.uk/catalogue/PUB19098/psyc-ther-ann-rep-2014–15.pdf. Accessed 4 2017.

Ilyas, S., & Moncrieff, J. (2012). Trends in prescriptions and costs of drugs for mental disorders in England, 1998–2010. *The British Journal of Psychiatry, 200,* 393–398.

Insel, T. (2013). *Director's blog: Transforming diagnosis.* National Institute of Mental Health. http://www.nimh.nih.gov/about/director/2013/transforming-diagnosis.shtml. Accessed 9 Apr 2015.

Insel, T. (2014). *Director's blog: A new approach to clinical trials.* National Institute of Mental Health. http://www.nimh.nih.gov/about/director/2014/a-new-approach-to-clinical-trials.shtml. Accessed 1 Feb 2015.

JAMA. (2016). *Journal of the American Medical Association,* vol. 315, n. 4; Michael, E. T. Recommendations for Screening for Depression in Adults, pp. 349–350; Howard, B., Fontanarosa, P. B. & Golub, R. M. JAMA Welcomes the US Preventive Services Task Force, pp. 351–352.

Kabat-Zinn, J. (1991). *Full catastrophe living: Using the wisdom of your body and mind to face stress, pain, and illness.* New York: Delta Trade Paperbacks.

Kabat-Zinn, J., Wheeler, E., Light, T., et al. (1998). Influence of a mindfulness meditation-based stress reduction intervention on rates of skin clearing in patients with moderate to severe psoriasis undergoing phototherapy (UVB) and photochemotherapy (PUVA). *Psychosomatic Medicine, 60*(5), 625–632.

Kassirer, J. P. (2005). *On the take: How medicine's complicity with big business can endanger your health.* Oxford: Oxford University Press.

Kramer, P. D. (2016). *Ordinarily well: The case for antidepressants.* New York: Farrar, Straus and Giroux.

Law, J. (2006). *Big pharma: How the world's biggest drug companies control illness.* London: Constable & Robinson Ltd.

Linde, K., Sigterman, K., Kriston, L., et al. (2015a). Effectiveness of psychological treatments for depressive disorders in primary care: Systematic review and meta-analysis. *Annals of Family Medicine, 13*(1), 56–68.

Linde, K., Kriston, L., Rücker, G., et al. (2015b). Efficacy and acceptability of pharmacological treatments for depressive disorders in primary care: Systematic review and network meta-analysis. *Annals of Family Medicine, 13*(1), 69–79.

Moynihan, R. (2003). The making of a disease: Female sexual dysfunction. *Britsh Medical Journal, 326*(7379), 45–47.

Moynihan, R. (2005). The marketing of a disease: Female sexual dysfunction. *Britsh Medical Journal, 330*(7484), 192–194.

Moynihan, R., & Cassels, A. (2005). *Selling sickness: How the world's biggest pharmaceutical companies are turning us all into patients.* Toronto: Greystone Books.

Moynihan, R., & Mintzes, B. (2010). *Sex, lies and pharmaceuticals: How drug companies plan to profit from female sexual dysfunction.* Toronto: Greystone Books.

NICE: National Institute for Health and Care Excellence. (2009). *Depression in adults: The treatment and management of depression in adults.* https://www.nice.org.uk/guidance/cg90. Accessed 12 Apr 2015.

Payer, L. (1992). *Disease-mongers: How doctors, drug companies, and insurers are making you feel sick.* New York: John Wiley.

Pratt, L. A., Brody, D. J., and Qiuping, G. U. (2011, October). Antidepressant use in persons aged 12 and over: United States, 2005–2008. NCHS Data Brief, No. 76, https://www.cdc.gov/nchs/data/databriefs/db76.pdf. Accessed 4 Jan 2017.

Reardon, S. (2014). NIH rethinks psychiatry trials. *Nature, 507*(7492), 288.

Richards, D., Ekers, D., & McMillan, D. A. (2016). Cost and outcome of behavioural activation versus cognitive behavioural therapy for depression (COBRA): A randomised, controlled, non-inferiority trial. *The Lancet, 388,* 871–880.

Shedler, J. (2010). The efficacy of psychodynamic psychotherapy. *American Psychology, 65*(2), 98–109.

Smith, R. (2006). *The trouble with medical journals*. London: The Royal Society of Medicine Press.

Spence, R., Roberts, A., Ariti, C., & Bardsley, M. (2014). *Focus on: Antidepressant prescribing. Trends in the prescribing of antidepressants in primary care*. Quality Watch, The Health Foundation, Nuffield Trust. http://www.health.org.uk/sites/health/files/QualityWatch_FocusOn AndidepressantPrescribing.pdf. Accessed 4 Jan 2017.

Stephenson, C. P., Karanges, E., & McGregor, I. S. (2013). Trends in the utilisation of psychotropic medications in Australia from 2000 to 2011. *Australian and New Zealand Journal of Psychiatry, 47*(1), 74–87. doi:10.1177/0004867412466595.

Talking Therapies. (2011). *Talking Therapies: A Four-year Plan of Action*. Department of Health. https://www.gov.uk/government/uploads/system/uploads/attachment_data/file/213765/dh_123985.pdf. Accessed 12 Apr 2015.

Tang, Y. Y., Tang, R., & Posner, M. I. (2013). Brief meditation training induces smoking reduction. *Proceedings of the National Academy of Sciences of the United States of America, 110*(34), 13971–13975.

The Guardian. (2013). *Peer review and scientific publishing. Nobel winner declares boycott of top science journals*. http://www.theguardian.com/science/2013/dec/09/nobel-winner-boycott-science-journals. Accessed 11 Apr 2015.

The Guardian. (2014, May 28). Rise in antidepressant prescriptions rates in England: Get the data. Ami Sedghi. https://www.theguardian.com/news/datablog/2014/may/28/rise-in-antidepressant-prescriptions-rates-in-england-get-the-data. Accessed 4 Jan 2017.

The Guardian. (2016, July 5). Mental health. Antidepressant prescriptions in England double in a decade. James Meikle. https://www.theguardian.com/society/2016/jul/05/antidepressant-prescriptions-in-england-double-in-a-decade. Accessed 4 Jan 2017.

The New York Review of Books. (2011a, June 23). The epidemic of mental illness: Why? Marcia Angell. http://www.nybooks.com/articles/2011/06/23/epidemic-mental-illness-why/. Accessed 4 Jan 2017.

The New York Review of Books. (2011b, July 14). The illusions of psychiatry. Marcia Angell. http://www.nybooks.com/articles/2011/07/14/illusions-of-psychiatry/. Accessed 4 Jan 2017.

Tone, A. (2009). *The age of anxiety: A history of America's turbulent affair with tranquilizers*. New York: Basic Books.

van Grieken, R. A., Kirkenier, A., Koeter, M., et al. (2014). Helpful self-management strategies to cope with enduring depression from the patients point of view: A concept map study. *BMC Psychiatry, 14*(331). doi:10.1186/s12888-014-0331-7.

Watters, E. (2010). *Crazy like us: The globalization of the American psyche.* New York: Free Press.

Whitfield, G., & Williams, C. (2003). The evidence base for cognitive—Behavioural therapy in depression: Delivery in busy clinical settings. *Advances in Psychiatric Treatment, 9,* 21–30.

Williams, M., Teasdale, J., & Segal, Z., et al. (2007). *The mindful way through depression: Freeing yourself from chronic unhappiness.* New York: The Guilford Press.

Wislar, J. S., Flanagin, A., & Fontanarosa, P. B., et al. (2011). Honorary and ghost authorship in high impact biomedical journals: A cross sectional survey. *British Medical Journal, 343*: d6128.

Appendix

A series of conferences were organised between April and June 2014 by the University of Trieste, together with the local national healthcare service, the Azienda per l'Assistenza Sanitaria n° 1 Triestina, at the university campus in the former San Giovanni Psychiatric Hospital. Highly qualified researchers showed the results gained by the UK National Health Service (NHS) when it applied the National Institute for Care and Clinical Excellence (NICE) guidelines about the most appropriate treatment for depression. The titles and speakers were:

PHARMAGEDDON. David Healy, Professor of Psychiatry and Director of the North Wales Department of Psychological Medicine, Cardiff University, UK.

STEPPING INTO A NEW WORLD OF LOW INTENSITY PSYCHOTHERAPY. David Richards, Professor of Mental Health Services Research and NIHR Senior Investigator, University of Exeter Medical School, UK.

SLOW MEDICINE. Gianfranco Domenighetti, Professore presso l'Università della Svizzera Italiana di Lugano, CH: Andrea Gardini, **Direttore** Sanitario dell'Azienda Ospedaliero, Universitaria di Ferrara.

© The Editor(s) (if applicable) and The Author(s) 2017
T. Giraldi, *Unhappiness, Sadness and 'Depression'*,
DOI 10.1007/978-3-319-57657-2

DOES PSYCHOPHARMACOLOGY HAVE A FUTURE? Nikolas Rose, Professor of Sociology, Head of the Department of Social Science, Health and Medicine, King's College, London, UK.

The video recording of the conference, including an introduction and discussion, is available at:
https://www.youtube.com/channel/UCZfh9yTuav_RZv69TCQgGpg.
Further updates about the problems of treating depression are available at the author's website:
http://www.tulliogiraldi.it/it_IT/.

Bibliography

Ashton Keller, A., Hamer, R., & Rosen, R. C. (1997). Serotonin reuptake inhibitor-induced sexual dysfunction and its treatment: A large-scale retrospective study of 596 psychiatric outpatients. *Journal of Sex and Marital Therapy, 23*(3), 165–175.

Balon, R. (2006). SSRI-associated sexual dysfunction. *American Journal of Psychiatry, 163*(9), 1504–1509.

Council for International Organizations of Medical Sciences. (2002). *International Ethical Guidelines for Biomedical Research Involving Human Subjects.* Accessed March 14, 2014, from http://www.cioms.ch/publications/layout_guide2002.pdf.

Cusack, B., Nelson, A., & Richelson, E. (1994). Binding of antidepressants to human brain receptors: Focus on newer generation compounds. *Psychopharmacology, 114*(4), 559–565.

DeVane, C. L. (2006). Antidepressant–drug interactions are potentially but rarely clinically significant. *Neuropsychopharmacology, 31*(8), 1594–1604.

Fava, M., & Rankin, M. R. (2002). Sexual functioning and SSRIs. *Journal of Clinical Psychiatry, 60*(5), 13–16.

Field, T. (2010). Prenatal depression and selective serotonin reuptake inhibitors. *International Journal of Neurosciences, 120*(3), 163–167.

Friedman, R. A. (2014). Antidepressants' black-box warning-10 years later. *New England Journal of Medicine, 371*(18), 1666–1668.

© The Editor(s) (if applicable) and The Author(s) 2017
T. Giraldi, *Unhappiness, Sadness and 'Depression'*,
DOI 10.1007/978-3-319-57657-2

Friedman, R. A., & Leon, A. C. (2007). Expanding the black box—Depression, antidepressants, and the risk of suicide. *New England Journal of Medicine, 356*(23), 2343–2346.

Haddad, P. (1998). The SSRI discontinuation syndrome. *Journal of Psychopharmacology, 12*(3), 305–313.

Hall, W. D. (2006). How have the SSRI antidepressants affected suicide risk? *Lancet, 367*(9527), 1959–1962.

Hawton, K., Casañas, I., Comabella, C., & Saunders, K. (2013). Risk factors for suicide in individuals with depression: A systematic review. *Journal of Affective Disorders, 147*(1–3), 17–28.

Healy, D., & Leonard, B. E. (1987). Monoamine transport in depression: Kinetics and dynamics. *Journal of Affective Disorders, 12*(2), 91–103.

Hemeryck, A., & Belpaire, F. M. (2002). Selective serotonin reuptake inhibitors and cytochrome P-450 mediated drug–drug interactions: An update. *Current Drug Metabolism, 3*(1), 13–37.

Jablensky, A. (1999). The nature of psychiatric classification: Issues beyond ICD-10 and DSM-IV. *Australian and New Zeland Journal of Psychiatry, 33*(2), 137–144.

JAMA PATIENT PAGE | Preventive *Medicine screening for depression. Depression is a type of mental illness that often goes unrecognized and untreated,* 428; Siu, A.L. and the US Preventive Services Task Force (USPSTF). *Screening for depression in adults. US Preventive services task force recommendation statement,* 380–387.

Kennedy, S. H., & Rizvi, S. (2009). Sexual dysfunction, depression, and the impact of antidepressants. *Journal of Clinical Psychopharmacology, 29*(2), 157–164.

Khan, A., Faucett, J., Lichtenberg, P., Kirsch, I., & Brown W.A. (2012). A systematic review of comparative efficacy of treatments and controls for depression. *PLoS ONE, 7*(7), e41778.

Leucht, S., Hierl, S., Kissling, W., Dold M., & Davis J. M. (2012). Putting the efficacy of psychiatric and general medicine medication into perspective: Review of meta-analyses. *British Journal of Psychiatry, 200*(2), 97–106.

Ludwig, J., & Marcotte, D. E. (2005). Anti-depressants, suicide, and drug regulation. *Journal of Policy Analysis and Management, 24*(2), 249–272.

Mindfulness. (2015). *Publications.* Accessed April 16, 2015, from http://www.umassmed.edu/cfm/research/publications/.

Moncrieff, J. (2002, April 26). *Drug treatment in modern psychiatry:The history of a delusion. Talk given at critical psychiatry network conference, "Beyond drugs and custody: Renewing mental health practice".* Accessed March 20, 2015, from http://www.critpsynet.freeuk.com/Moncrieff.htm.

Moncrieff, J. (2007). *The myth of the chemical cure: A critique of psychiatric drug treatment.* Basingstoke: Palgrave Macmillan.

Nestler, E. J., Barrot, M., DiLeone, R. J., et al. (2002). Neurobiology of depression. *Neuron, 34*(1), 13–25.

Nielsen, M., Hansen, E. H., & Gøtzsche, P. C. (2012). What is the difference between dependence and withdrawal reactions? A comparison of benzodiazepines and selective serotonin re-uptake inhibitors. *Addiction, 107*(5), 900–908.

Prabhakar, D., & Balon, R. (2010). How do SSRIs cause sexual dysfunction. *Current Psychiatry, 9*(12), 30–35.

Scull, E. (2009). *Hysteria the disturbing history.* Oxford: Oxford University Press.

Serebruany, V. L. (2006). Selective serotonin reuptake inhibitors and increased bleeding risk: Are we missing something? *American Journal of Medicine, 119*(2), 113–116.

Sie, S. D., Wennink, J. M., van Driel, J. J., & van Weissenbruch, M. (2012). Maternal use of SSRIs, SNRIs and NaSSAs: Practical recommendations during pregnancy and lactation. *Archives of Disease in Childhood-Fetal and Neonatal Edition, 97*(6), F472–F476.

Stone, M. B. (2014). The FDA warning on antidepressants and suicidality—Why the controversy? *The New England Journal of Medicine, 371*(18), 1668–1671.

Tatsumi, M., Groshan, K., Blakely, R. D., & Richelson, E. (1997). Pharmacological profile of antidepressants and related compounds at human monoamine transporters. *European Journal of Pharmacology, 340*(2–3), 249–258.

Tone, A., & Siegel Watkins, E. (2007). *Medicating modern America: Prescription drugs in history.* New York: New York University Press.

Warner, C. H., Bobo, W., Warner, C., Reid S., & Rachal J, (2006). Antidepressant discontinuation syndrome. *American Family Physician, 74*(3), 449–456.

Weinrieb, R. M., Auriacombe, M., Lynch, K. G., & Lewis, J. D. (2005). Selective serotonin re-uptake inhibitors and the risk of bleeding. *Expert Opinion in Drug Safety, 4*(2), 337–344.

Whittington, C. J., Kendall, T., Fonagy, P., Cottrell, D., Cotgrove, A., & Boddington, E. (2004). Selective serotonin reuptake inhibitors in childhood depression: Systematic review of published versus unpublished data. *Lancet, 363*(9418), 1341–1345.

WHO. (2003). WHO expert committee on drug dependence: Thirty-third Report, 33. Accessed May 30, 2016, from http://apps.who.int/iris/bitstream/10665/42655/1/WHO_TRS_915.pdf.

Index

© The Editor(s) (if applicable) and The Author(s) 2017
T. Giraldi, *Unhappiness, Sadness and 'Depression'*,
DOI 10.1007/978-3-319-57657-2

The manufacturer's authorised representative in the EU is Springer
Nature Customer Service Centre GmbH, Europaplatz 3, 69115 Heidelberg,
Germany. If you have any concerns regarding our products, please
contact ProductSafety@springernature.com

Printed and bound by CPI Group (UK) Ltd, Croydon, CR0 4YY
27/04/2026
02097624-0001